Jaime L. Fridman MD

HYPERTENSION
A Practical Approach

HYPERTENSION
A Practical Approach

Edited by
Marvin Moser, M.D.
Clinical Professor of Medicine, New York Medical College; Physician-in-Charge, Hypertension Clinic, Westchester County Medical Center, Valhalla, New York; Chief of Cardiology, White Plains Hospital, White Plains, New York

Little, Brown and Company Boston

First Edition

Library of Congress catalog card No. 75–14873

ISBN 0316–58540–8

Printed in the United States of America

Preface

Twenty-four million Americans suffer from hypertension . . . most do not know they have it. Only one-eighth are receiving adequate therapy—this in the face of the fact that high blood pressure is the primary cause of 60,000 American deaths each year and is a significant causative factor in the more than 1,500,000 heart attacks and strokes suffered annually by Americans.

John Knowles, *Journal of Medical Education,* January, 1974

Recently several excellent texts that deal in depth with the subject of hypertension have been published. Great emphasis is placed upon mechanisms of hypertension and diagnosis in these books. We believe that a less complicated and more practical approach to the subject will be of use to the practicing physician, who does not always have time to delve deeply into a specific topic, yet wants to stay in touch with recent developments. With this in mind, we have written *Hypertension: A Practical Approach.*

Important basic data regarding the role of the kidney, salt, and plasma volume in experimental, as well as human, hypertension are presented. The role of the adrenal gland and renin in hypertension is also explored in some depth. The major emphasis of the book, however, is on the modern management and drug treatment of primary hypertension. We hope that it will be of value to the physician as he encounters the large number of hypertensive patients in his daily practice.

This book evolved from a symposium on hypertension which was held in Tarrytown, New York, in April, 1974, under the cosponsorship of the New York Medical College, the

Westchester Heart Association and the Westchester County Medical Society, and the Westchester Academy of Medicine, as part of the CIBA Pharmaceutical Medical Horizon Program. We are indebted to the USV Pharmaceutical Corporation for the title of the book.

M. M.

Introduction

Many physicians have heard a great deal about the subject of high blood pressure in recent years at local and national medical meetings, but despite this emphasis, *major* changes in treatment patterns have only recently begun to occur. Thus far we have failed to make a significant impact on this major cardiovascular disease risk factor, hypertension.

The first reason for our failure to meet the challenge of hypertension stems from the fact that medical students, interns, residents, and practicing physicians had been taught for years that hypertension was "benign," was only a symptom, and, since little was known about it, need not be taken seriously —this, despite good insurance data to the contrary. We had no simple or specific therapy before the 1940s anyway, so before that time the attitude was why treat if the treatment was complicated and frequently produced severe morbidity? It was not until definitive studies—which Dr. Stamler describes clearly in Chapter 1—demonstrated that hypertension was indeed a serious risk factor in heart disease, strokes, and progressive kidney failure that these myths of yesteryear were refuted.

The second reason for our failure to meet the challenge is that hypertension is frequently asymptomatic and is not a dramatic disease until a serious complication occurs. Even with appropriate therapy available, physicians have frequently been loath to start therapy that might produce symptoms in patients who otherwise felt well. Until recent years, there were no definitive data that the long-term treatment of mild to moderately severe or asymptomatic hypertension was beneficial. Now that such information is available, the risk of producing some side effects in some patients is clearly justifiable.

The third reason for our failure may relate to the fact that hypertension remains an enigma. Physicians, as scientists, do not like to treat an entity that they do not understand. For the past 15–20 years, millions of dollars have been spent on research aimed at discovering the mechanism or mechanisms of this disease. Much effort has gone into the training of physicians in the performance of tests, and many thousands of people have been investigated for treatable forms of hypertension. Despite all this effort, less than 5 percent of patients with high blood pressure have been found with a secondary cause: less than 2–3 percent have been found to have renovascular diseases; 1–2 percent, an aldosterone-secreting tumor; and the remaining 1 percent, coarctation of the aorta, pheochromocytoma, and various endocrinopathies. *We have hospitalized too many patients and made the work-up of hypertension a complicated, often mysterious procedure.* The physician has attended meetings where new tests or new complicated ways of doing old tests are described. He has returned to his practice feeling guilty that he is not equipped or able to do these tests and perhaps not sophisticated enough to know when to do them. Mechanisms rather than treatment have been stressed. The exciting or esoteric has been highlighted.

All of this effort has not been wasted. Much has been learned about the roles of aldosterone and renin and neurogenic factors in hypertension, and these facts may someday lead to a real understanding and a more exacting approach to treatment. Basic research in all of these areas must continue; however, using the knowledge already at hand, we must place a greater emphasis on simplifying our approach to diagnosis and treatment if we are to alter the status of this "reversible" risk factor as one of our most important unsolved public health problems.

Table 1 summarizes data from an audit of 80 hospitals, both teaching and nonteaching, that have recently been surveyed. These data show that less than 30 percent of over 8,000 patients with a diastolic blood pressure on admission of 100 mm Hg or more were listed on the discharge sheet as having hypertension. Less than one-third received diuretic therapy, and less

Table 1. Patients with Diastolic Blood Pressure of 100 mm Hg or over, 80 United States PAS Hospitals by Teaching Status, July–September, 1972

Hospital Type	Number of Patients with Diastolic Blood Pressure of 100 mm Hg or over	Percent with Record of		
		Hyper-tension Diagnosis	Diuretics	Specific Antihyper-tensives
All Hospitals	8,524	27	32	17
Nonteaching	3,827	26	31	18
Teaching	4,697	28	33	17

From Commission on Professional and Hospital Activities. *Professional Activity Study,* Vol. II, No. 19. Ann Arbor, Mich., Dec., 1973.

than 20 percent received specific antihypertensive drugs. Data from the nonteaching hospitals are approximately the same as that from the teaching institutions. Other studies have demonstrated identical findings. These figures are not from 1965 (before the recent emphasis on hypertension); they are from 1972. Physicians apparently have not yet responded to data that are available—namely, that hypertension is prevalent, that hypertension is serious, that hypertension can be controlled, and that some of its serious complications can be prevented.

Contents

Contributing Authors

Ray W. Gifford, Jr., M.D.
Head, Department of Hypertension and Nephrology, The Cleveland Clinic Foundation, Cleveland

J. Caulie Gunnells, Jr., M.D.
Professor of Medicine, Department of Medicine, Division of Nephrology, Duke University School of Medicine, Durham, North Carolina

Arthur H. Hayes, Jr., M.D.
Associate Professor of Medicine and Pharmacology, and Chief, Division of Clinical Pharmacology, The Pennsylvania State University College of Medicine, The Milton S. Hershey Medical Center, Hershey

William L. McGuffin, Jr., M.D.
Fellow, Department of Medicine, Division of Nephrology, Duke University School of Medicine, Durham, North Carolina

Marvin Moser, M.D.
Clinical Professor of Medicine, New York Medical College; Physician-in-Charge, Hypertension Clinic, Westchester County Medical Center, Valhalla, New York; Chief of Cardiology, White Plains Hospital, White Plains, New York

Jeremiah Stamler, M.D.
Professor and Chairman, Department of Community Health and Preventive Medicine, Northwestern University Medical School; Chairman, Department of Community Health and Preventive Medicine, Northwestern Memorial Hospital, Chicago

Louis Tobian, M.D.
Professor of Medicine, Department of Medicine, University of Minnesota Medical School; Head, Hypertension-Renal Section, University of Minnesota Hospital, Minneapolis

HYPERTENSION
A Practical Approach

Notice

The indications and dosages of all drugs in this manual have been recommended in the medical literature and conform to the practices of the general medical community. The medications described do not necessarily have specific approval by the Food and Drug Administration for use in the diseases and dosages for which they are recommended. The package insert for each drug should be consulted for use and dosage as approved by the FDA. Because standards for usage change, it is advisable to keep abreast of revised recommendations, particularly those concerning new drugs.

1. Epidemiology of Hypertension: Achievements and Challenges

Jeremiah Stamler

Hypertensive Disease as a Mass Public Health Problem

One of the major achievements of cardiovascular epidemiology in recent years is the accumulation of data on populations, which unequivocally point to hypertensive disease as a mass public health problem in the United States—one of the most prevalent and important afflictions producing premature sickness, disability, and death in our adult population.

The data collected a decade ago on a random sample of the United States adult population ages 18–79 by the National Health Examination Survey of the Public Health Service [1, 2] indicate that about 15 percent of whites and 28 percent of blacks have high blood pressure. These estimates are based on World Health Organization criteria for hypertension: systolic $\geqq$ 160 mm Hg and/or diastolic $\geqq$ 95 mm Hg (Table 1-1).

As the accompanying data make clear, high blood pressure afflicts not only the elderly, but also young and middle-aged adults. At ages 25–34, 3.7 percent of white men, 12.5 percent of black men, 2.3 percent of white women, and 8.5 percent of black women are hypertensive (Table 1-1). The incidence rises steadily with age. At all ages up to 80, the incidence of hypertension is higher for blacks than for whites. Overall, the ratio is about 2:1, with twice as high a prevalence for blacks as for whites. Further, hypertension, when present, tends to be more severe in blacks than in whites. The disease is widespread among all strata of the adult population and in all geographic areas. It occurs in the low, middle, and upper income groups; in the North, East, South, and West; in people of all educa-

Table 1-1. Percentage of White and Negro Adults with Blood Pressures of at Least 160 mm Hg Systolic or 95 mm Hg Diastolic, by Sex and Age, United States, 1960–1962

Sex and Age	Systolic at Least 160 mm Hg		Diastolic at Least 95 mm Hg		Systolic at Least 160 mm Hg or Diastolic 95 mm Hg	
	White	Negro	White	Negro	White	Negro
Both sexes						
18–79 years	10.5	18.8	8.7	22.0	14.7	27.6
Men						
Total: 18–79 years	8.6	16.8	9.1	22.6	13.6	27.6
18–24 years	0.2	–	1.7	1.9	1.7	1.9
25–34 years	0.7	4.6	3.4	11.5	3.7	12.5
35–44 years	3.9	16.2	10.9	25.9	11.8	26.5
45–54 years	8.7	10.8	13.8	29.5	17.3	30.8
55–64 years	15.9	29.4	11.9	31.6	21.4	44.6
65–74 years	26.1	63.2	12.3	40.5	27.3	66.0
75–79 years	39.1	59.8	13.3	21.2	40.2	59.8
Women						
Total: 18–79 years	12.3	20.4	8.3	21.5	15.6	27.6
18–24 years	–	0.7	0.8	3.4	0.8	3.4
25–34 years	0.7	3.4	2.1	8.5	2.3	8.5
35–44 years	2.3	14.3	5.3	24.1	6.2	25.6
45–54 years	10.7	30.8	10.9	34.3	15.5	41.9
55–64 years	25.3	33.8	16.4	36.7	31.0	41.0
65–74 years	45.4	68.5	17.9	32.1	48.6	71.0
75–79 years	42.7	69.4	12.0	26.3	44.9	69.4

From U.S. Department of Health, Education, and Welfare [1].

tional levels; in residents of central metropolises and their suburbs, of small cities, and of rural areas.

Data consistent with these National Health Examination Survey estimates have been reported time and again by local surveys [3, 4]. The recent findings of the Chicago Heart Asso-

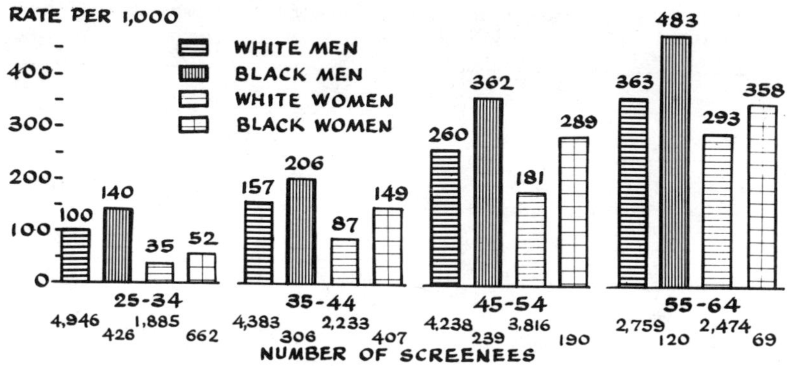

FIG. 1-1. Prevalence of high blood pressure by age, sex, and race. Criterion: systolic blood pressure ≧ 160 and/or diastolic blood pressure ≧ 95 mm Hg. Rates age-adjusted by five-year age groups to corresponding sex-race group in United States population, 1960. (From Stamler [4].)

ciation Detection Project in Industry, collected from 1967 to 1972 on approximately 40,000 employees of almost 100 companies, are typical (Figure 1-1) [5].

Further data along these lines are now becoming available from the massive screening efforts of the Hypertension Detection and Follow-up Program of the National Heart and Lung Institute, encompassing surveys of over 170,000 persons aged 30–69 in 14 communities across the country.

A sound current estimate is that 20 to 25 million Americans have elevated blood pressures. About twice as many blacks as whites have diastolic pressures of 90 mm Hg and greater. The relative rate is 3.3 times as high for black men as compared with white men at diastolic levels of 115 mm or higher and 5.6 times as high for black women as compared with white women.

Among young, middle-aged, and elderly adults with hypertension—men and women, white and black—a high proportion have evidence of cardiac involvement, that is, hypertensive heart disease (Table 1-2) [1, 2]. Not only is their blood pressure abnormally high, but medical examination also reveals

Table 1-2. Prevalence of Definite and Suspect Hypertensive Heart Disease for White and Negro Adults, by Age and Sex, United States, 1960–1962

	Men		Women	
Age	White	Negro	White	Negro
	Percent of Specified Population Group			
Definite hypertensive heart disease				
Total 18–79 years	6.5	19.1	9.8	22.2
18–24 years	0.2	1.9	–	1.6
25–34 years	1.1	5.2	0.7	4.7
35–44 years	4.0	15.2	2.7	14.0
45–54 years	7.7	24.4	6.8	31.5
55–64 years	11.7	33.1	19.5	46.4
65–74 years	16.3	50.2	37.5	66.4
75–79 years	24.0	32.3	37.1	69.5
Suspect hypertensive heart disease				
Total 18–79 years	5.0	7.6	3.3	4.7
18–24 years	1.5	1.5	–	–
25–34 years	1.2	7.3	0.7	–
35–44 years	4.0	6.2	0.8	3.6
45–54 years	4.3	10.5	3.4	5.9
55–64 years	7.3	13.8	8.5	15.0
65–74 years	13.8	–	8.4	10.3
75–79 years	15.7	21.4	10.7	14.2

From U.S. Department of Health, Education, and Welfare [1].

evidence of cardiac abnormalities, that is, on the electrocardiogram, or chest x-ray film, or both, even though the person often is still free of symptoms. When the disease has gone this far, risks of serious sickness, disability, and death are even greater than when elevated blood pressure is present without evidence of heart disease.

In keeping with the tendency for the prevalence of hypertension to be not only higher, but also more severe among blacks than whites, hypertensive heart disease is present at rates three, four, seven, and even nine times greater for blacks of a given age-sex group compared with whites of the same age-sex group (Table 1-2).

Hypertension as a Major Risk Factor for Cardiovascular Morbidity, Disability, and Mortality

Hypertensive disease is a serious mass public health problem, even though at any given time a majority of hypertensive persons are symptom-free. People with hypertension are at increased risk of experiencing major morbid cardiovascular events (especially heart failure, heart attack, stroke, and kidney failure), with resultant chronic illness and disability. Moreover, young and middle-aged adults with hypertension are at a markedly increased risk of dying prematurely from cardiovascular complications. This is true even for persons with only slight elevations of blood pressure. (The terms *mild* and *benign hypertension* are misleading and disarming and have blocked proper understanding of the seriousness of the problem both among the general public and among health professionals, including physicians.) For decades the insurance industry tried to drive home this point, with only limited success. The Society of Actuaries' most recent (1959) study clearly demonstrates the increased risk of premature death for persons with mild or moderate hypertension [6]. For example, it was found that men aged 35 with a blood pressure reading of 142/90 mm Hg *without any concomitant impairments,* experienced a survival rate of 80.6 percent over the next 20 years, compared with a survival rate of 89.0 percent for normotensive standard risks. That is, this "modest" elevation of blood pressure, which is all too frequently treated as insignificant and ignored by clinicians, was associated with a 76.4 percent higher mortality rate in middle age (19.4 percent versus 11.0 percent).

In recent years, this whole matter has been further clarified through the efforts of the major prospective epidemiologic research studies carried out in various parts of the United States. Figures 1-2 and 1-3 present the combined findings of five of these investigations working together in the national cooperative Pooling Project, namely, the Albany civil servant, the Chicago Peoples Gas Company, Chicago Western Electric Company, Framingham community, and Minneapolis–St. Paul business and professional men's studies [7]. These data are from 7,581 white men aged 30–59 at first examination. After exclusion of men with definite coronary heart disease, they

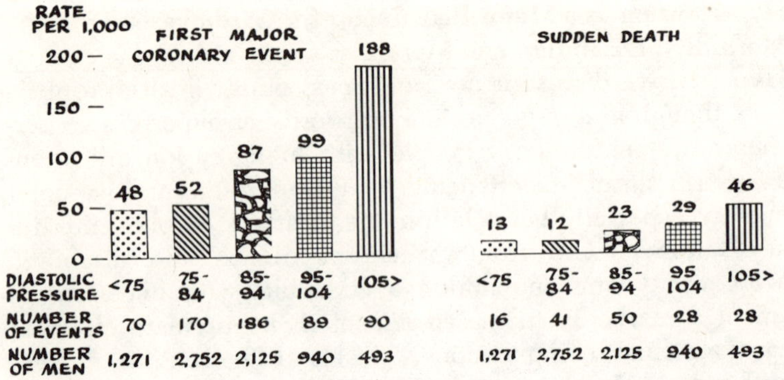

FIG. 1-2. National cooperative Pooling Project. Diastolic blood pressure level at beginning of study and 10-year age-adjusted rates per 1,000 men for first major coronary event and sudden death. First major coronary event includes nonfatal myocardial infarction, fatal myocardial infarction, sudden death due to coronary heart disease; U.S. white males aged 30–59 at beginning of study; all rates age-adjusted by 10-year age groups to the United States white male population, 1960. (From Inter-Society Commission for Heart Disease Resources [7].)

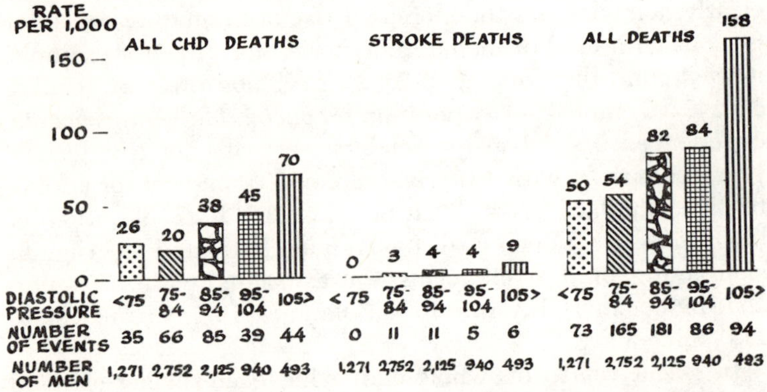

FIG. 1-3. National cooperative Pooling Project. Diastolic blood pressure level at beginning of study and 10-year age-adjusted rates per 1,000 men for any coronary death, stroke death, and death from all causes; United States white males aged 30–59 at beginning of study; all rates age-adjusted by 10-year age groups to the United States white male population, 1960. (From Inter-Society Commission for Heart Disease Resources [7].)

were classified on the basis of their diastolic blood pressure level at this single point in time. Diastolic blood pressure levels in the range of 95–104 mm Hg were recorded for 940 of these men (12.4 percent); another 493 (6.5 percent) had levels of 105 mm Hg or greater. Note that mortality over the next 10 years from heart attack, including sudden death, was twice as high in the group with so-called mild hypertension (diastolic levels of 95–104 mm Hg) compared with those who had normal diastolic pressures. Further, the increase in the risk of death from coronary disease, including sudden death, was more than threefold for the group of 493 men with pressures of 105 mm Hg and greater. The ten-year mortality from all causes was 60 percent higher for men with diastolic pressures 95–104 mm Hg, compared with those who were normotensive; it was 200 percent higher for those with diastolic pressures of 105 mm Hg or more. Note also the 60 percent greater mortality from all causes, compared to normotensives, even for the men with diastolic pressures of 85–94 mm Hg. These increases in risk for hypertensive persons persist at least up to age 65. Data on elderly people, available from at least one study, indicate that this conclusion may be true up to age 75 and even beyond.

Two other very important points are demonstrated by this group of studies. First, the effect of hypertension on risk is not artifactual; that is, it is not due to other risk factors but is a valid independent effect. Second, when hypertension coexists with other major risk factors (e.g., cigarette smoking, hypercholesterolemia), the risks are additive (Figs. 1-4 and 1-5). Thus, men who were aged 30–59 when first observed and in whom hypertension was the only risk factor, experienced twice as high a death rate over the next 10 years as men with no risk factors. When hypertension coexisted either with cigarette smoking or with hypercholesterolemia, the risk of dying was more than trebled. And when hypertension was present along with *both* these factors, the death rate was five times higher. These data practically speak for themselves in terms of their implications for public health and medical practice.

A *single blood pressure recorded* in a routine school examination of college entrants (young men in their late teens) has been found to be very meaningful in terms of prognosis [8]. Even that early in life, slight blood pressure elevation identifies people at greater risk. The data are from a study by Paffenbarger of men who were students at the University of Pennsylvania and Harvard University 20, 30, 40, or more years ago. First, he gathered data from the records of their college

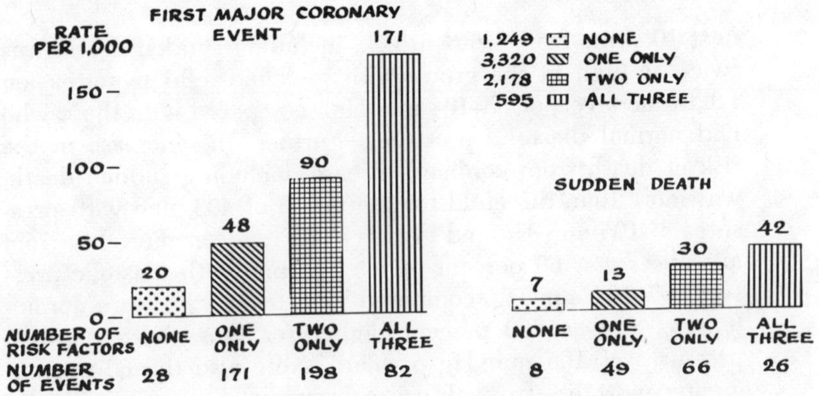

FIG. 1-4. National cooperative Pooling Project. Hypercholesterolemia, hypertension, cigarette smoking, and 10-year age-adjusted rates per 1,000 men for first major coronary event and sudden death. First major coronary event includes non-fatal myocardial infarction, fatal myocardial infarction, and sudden death due to coronary heart disease; United States white males aged 30–59 at beginning of study. All rates age-adjusted by 10-year age groups to the United States white male population, 1960. Cutting points: serum cholesterol ≧ 250 mg/dl; diastolic blood pressure ≧ 90 mm Hg; any use of cigarettes at beginning of study. (From Inter-Society Commission for Heart Disease Resources [7].)

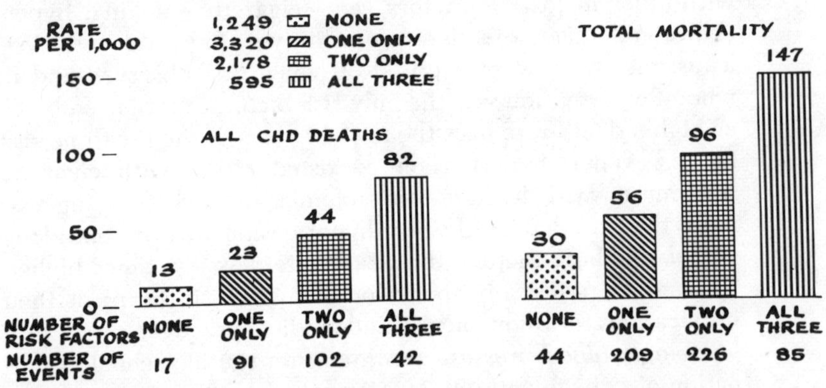

FIG. 1-5. National cooperative Pooling Project. Hypercholesterolemia, hypertension, cigarette smoking, and 10-year age-adjusted rates per 1,000 men for any coronary death and death from all causes; United States white males aged 30–59 at entry; all rates age-adjusted by 10-year age groups to the United States white male population, 1960. Cutting points: serum cholesterol ≧ 250 mg/dl; diastolic blood pressure ≧ 90 mm Hg; any use of cigarettes at beginning of study. (From Inter-Society Commission for Heart Disease Resources [7].)

entrance physical examinations. He then traced these people and determined who had died and the cause of death in each case and who was currently alive. Findings in the college examinations were studied for correlation with mortality. Systolic pressure at college entry was one of the variables Paffenbarger evaluated, and it was evaluated in a simple way, namely, as 130 mm Hg and above, or under 130 mm Hg. Consider the limitations of this set of data: a single measurement, time of day unknown, relation to meals unknown, relation to smoking unknown, examiner unknown, position unknown (lying, standing, or sitting)—a motley collection of unstandardized one-time measurements. *Yet the teen-age men with systolic pressures of 130 and above had a 1.6 times higher mortality from coronary disease over the next decades, compared with those whose pressures were under 130. This is a 60 percent higher mortality.*

These data also permit another look at *the combined effect on mortality of elevated blood pressure and cigarette smoking.* Like elevated blood pressure, smoking alone was associated with a 60 percent increase in risk. College entrants with a systolic blood pressure of 130 or above who were smoking 10 or more cigarettes a day experienced a 110 percent increase in risk of coronary death. The effects of the two risk factors are additive. The hypertensive person who smokes cigarettes is at greater risk than the hypertensive person who does not.

The implications of these data are self-evident and need to be acted on. Along with detection, *mass public education is sorely needed,* proceeding continuously and vigorously, not only among adults, but also among our youth. Efforts along these lines have in fact been undertaken recently. One example is the Chicago Heart Association's effort, both in industry and in high schools, to find those seriously endangered by blood pressure elevation, as well as by cigarette smoking, gross obesity, and hypercholesterolemia.

When the person with elevated blood pressure also has signs of hypertensive heart disease, the risks of morbidity and mortality are especially high. Our findings in the Peoples Gas Company study [9] are typical in this regard (Table 1-3). Note that for the 128 men with hypertensive heart disease, definite or suspect, mortality from all causes over 12 years

Table 1-3. Hypertension, Hypertensive Heart Disease, and Risk of Death, Cohort of 1,465 men aged 40–59 in 1958 (Peoples Gas Company Study, 1958–1970)

		12-Year Age-Adjusted Mortality Rate per 1,000				
1958 Findings	Number of Men	All Causes	All CVR	Sudden Death	Myocardial Infarction	Stroke
No organ system abnormalities, none of three risk factors	208	70	8	0	8	0
No organ system abnormalities, hypertensive	147	156	53	22	30	12
Suspect hypertensive heart disease	53	268	159	57	117	21
Definite hypertensive heart disease	75	385	309	142	158	99

From Stamler, J., Berkson, D. M., and Lindberg, H. A. In Wissler, R. W., and Geer, J. C. (Eds.), *Pathogenesis of Atherosclerosis.* Williams & Wilkins, Baltimore, © 1972, American Association of Pathologists and Bacteriologists.

of follow-up was almost five times as high as for the group of 208 men at lowest risk, with most of the excess deaths due to cardiovascular causes. Note also that in this cohort of middle-aged employed men, over 90 percent of whom were white and, at entry into this study, free of evidence of definite coronary heart disease, 128 of 275 hypertensive men (46.5 percent) showed evidence of hypertensive heart disease. As previously noted, this proportion is even higher in the general population, white and black, but especially the latter. To repeat: National Health Examination Survey data indicates that in 1960–1962 there were about 12 million white and 3 million black adults aged 18–79 with definite or suspect hypertensive heart disease, or a total of 15 million. These numbers are undoubtedly greater today, constituting a huge pool of people with markedly increased risk of mortality, including premature mortality (e.g., before age 65).

Table 1-4. Social Security Disability Data, United States, 1969

Cause of Disability	White Male		White Female		Black Male		Black Female	
	Number	Percent	Number	Percent	Number	Percent	Number	Percent
All causes	218,188	100.0	76,203	100.0	33,233	100.0	13,286	100.0
Circulatory diseases	69,435	31.8	19,739	25.9	10,502	31.6	5,226	39.3
Musculoskeletal diseases	27,375	12.5	13,619	17.9	4,100	17.9	1,760	13.2
Mental disease	25,743	11.8	11,097	14.6	4,394	13.2	1,333	10.0
Neoplastic diseases	21,954	10.1	9,926	13.0	2,356	7.1	1,215	9.1
Respiratory disease	17,956	8.2	3,123	4.1	1,516	4.6	485	3.7
Accidents	19,942	9.1	4,257	5.6	3,342	10.1	463	3.5
Other diseases	35,783	16.4	14,442	19.0	7,023	21.1	2,804	21.1

From Lerner [10].

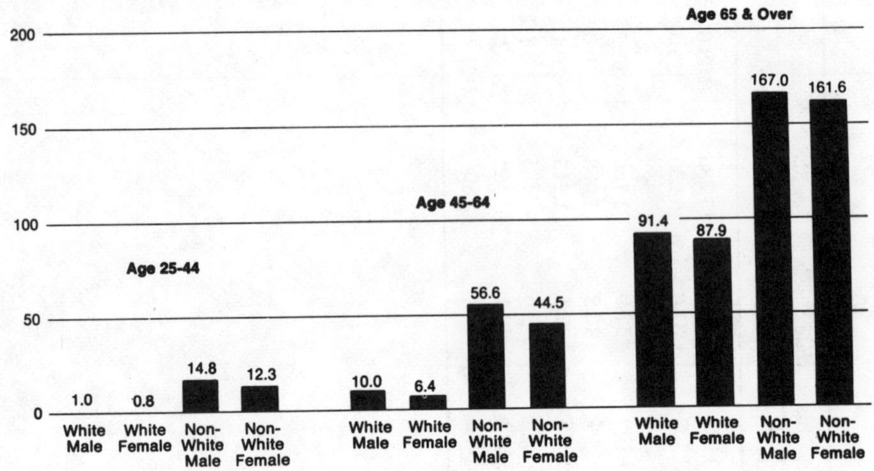

FIG. 1-6. Hypertensive disease mortality rates by age, sex, and race, United States, 1969 (per 100,000 population). (From American Heart Association [11]. © 1972, American Heart Association, Inc., reprinted with permission.)

Increased mortality is not the only problem. As data from the Social Security Administration clearly shows, a sizable amount of disability in the labor force—at a great economic cost to the workers involved, to society, and to government—is attributable to hypertensive disease (Table 1-4) [10]. Overall, of the 340,910 worker disability allowances in 1969, which is the year of latest record, 31 percent were due to diseases of the circulatory system, which was at the top of the list for each of the four major sex-race groups. Conservatively, in at least one-third, hypertension was a major contributing cause of their disabling illness. Therefore, hypertensive disease and its complications rank high on the list as producers of disability for all of the major sex-race groups in the labor force, taking a disproportionate toll among blacks, as expected in view of their prevalence rates for hypertensive disease in general and hypertensive heart disease in particular.

Finally, to round out this account of the impact of hypertensive disease on health, the overall vital statistics on mortality from *hypertensive disease* merit citation (Fig. 1-6) [11]. For all four major sex-race groups, mortality rises with age.

Table 1-5. Percentage Decrease in Death Rate for Hypertensive Disease, 1940–1960, by Age, Color, and Sex, United States (ICD Codes 440–447, 7th Revision)

Age	White		Nonwhite	
	Male	Female	Male	Female
All ages, age-adjusted	59.7	62.8	37.9	40.6
25–34	67.7	81.2	33.3	48.3
35–44	68.3	83.9	34.5	55.2
45–54	65.3	75.9	45.7	53.3
55–64	61.8	69.4	35.0	37.4
65–74	60.7	63.4	32.7	33.8
75–84	57.4	56.3	44.5	27.5
85 and over	49.6	45.3	30.2	25.1

From Moriyama, I. M., Krueger, D. E., and Stamler, J. *Cardiovascular Diseases in the United States*. Harvard University Press, Cambridge, Mass., © 1971 by the President and Fellows of Harvard College.

At all ages (this is true up to age 85) the rate for nonwhites, i.e., blacks, is much higher than for whites: for males aged 25–44, 14.8 versus 1.0; for females of this age, 12.3 versus 0.8. At ages 45–64, the mortality rates for blacks is six and seven times as high as for whites, for men and women respectively.* Mortality for cerebrovascular disease shows very similar patterns, reflecting the fact that *hypertension is the single most important risk factor for strokes, both atherothrombotic (occlusive) and hemorrhagic.*

The data in Figure 1-6 are for 1969, the year of latest record. Statistics are also available by age, sex, and race for the trend of mortality for hypertensive disease for the period 1940–1960 (Table 1-5) [12]. The trend for white men and women was steadily downward throughout this period, with a steeper rate of decline beginning early in the 1950s. Maximum decreases were for the 35–44 age group: 68 and 84 percent for white men and white women, respectively. At all ages up to 65, the decline in rate was considerably greater for women than for men.

* While these statistics give a qualitatively valid insight into the impact of hypertensive disease on mortality, they are quantitatively misleading, i.e., they underestimate badly, due to problems in death certification and coding.

Comparison of the rates for 1969 makes it clear that this downward trend continued during the 1960s.

The long-term decline in hypertensive disease mortality was greater for whites than for blacks during this period, and this phenomenon certainly is another serious challenge. As a result of these trends, the mortality ratio of blacks to whites for hypertensive disease increased substantially over the past 20 years.

Considerable evidence is available indicating that the observed decline in mortality for hypertensive disease in general was real. The causes and reasons for the lesser decline for males than for females and for nonwhites than for whites remain obscure.

Introduction of effective pharmacologic agents for the lowering of blood pressure has been implicated as a possible factor responsible for the decline in mortality for hypertensive disease in general. However, these drugs cannot account for the sizable 1940–1950 downward trend exhibited by white males and white females, since modern antihypertensive medication dates from 1950. It is more likely that a secular trend has occurred, largely independent of the effects of the new antihypertensive drugs. This hypothesis is supported by the findings of recent population surveys, which will be discussed subsequently, showing that in a large proportion of persons with hypertension, the condition is undetected and undiagnosed, often for many years, that a large proportion of persons with known hypertension are not on any treatment, and that a large proportion of those under treatment continue to have elevated blood pressures. Thus, only a small minority of persons with hypertension are actually receiving effective long-term therapy. Therefore, it is a moot question whether or not the limited application of modern treatment is sufficient in scope and impact to account even partially for the observed downward trend in hypertensive disease mortality since 1950.

Effective Medication

One of the major achievements of the past 20 years is the development of drugs for the treatment of hypertension, the demonstration of their optimal usage (often in combination), and their efficacy in preventing morbidity, disability, and mortality.

Many physicians are old enough to have painful memories of the situation before 1950, when, in desperation, hypertensive people were given large doses of barbiturates or subjected to major surgery or drastic dietary restrictions, often with only limited benefit. Now, many types of effective antihypertensive medications are available, and painstaking research has elucidated the maximum benefit-to-risk ratios with judicious combinations of these drugs. The massive amount of information being accumulated on thousands of patients by the national cooperative Hypertension Detection and Follow-up Program of the National Heart and Lung Institute is confirming that blood pressures in a sizable proportion of persons with less severe elevations can be normalized with a single medication, particularly an oral diuretic. It is also refining a system of long-term treatment, epitomized by the term *stepped care* (i.e., over weeks and months), which involves progressive addition and adjustment of combinations of drugs and their dosage to achieve sustained normalization of blood pressure in a high percentage of patients with more severe hypertension. This type of research may be viewed by some as unexciting, but without these patient, long-term efforts, we would be in no position to talk about the large-scale control of this disease.

The kind of therapeutic effect that can be obtained with antihypertensive medication is illustrated in Table 1-6, from the Veterans Administration Cooperative Study Group on Antihypertensive Agents [13, 14]. As is evident, men given placebo experienced virtually no reduction in pressure. The effect of an active drug combination was clear-cut: There was an average reduction of about 30 mm Hg in systolic pressure and about 16 mm Hg in diastolic pressure in men with average diastolic pressures at entry into the study in the range of 90–114 mm Hg. Even greater average declines occurred in men with severe hypertension (average baseline diastolic pressures of 115–129 mm Hg) (Table 1-6). These decreases were accomplished using the combination of thiazide, reserpine, and hydralazine. Details of patient management with these drugs will be discussed in Chapter 5.

Table 1-6. Effectiveness of Antihypertensive Treatment in Lowering Diastolic Pressure, Veterans Administration Cooperative Study Group on Antihypertensive Agents

	Average Diastolic Pressure (mm Hg) in Men Originally 115–129 mm Hg	
	Control (Placebo)	Treated
Start of study	121.0	121.2
At 4 months	118.5	93.1
At 12 months	118.8	91.6
At 24 months	119.7	91.5

From Freis et al. *J. A. M. A.*, Dec. 11, 1967, Vol. 202, p. 1028. Copyright 1967 American Medical Association.

This excellent effect on blood pressure deserves special emphasis in view of the extensive evidence indicating that the majority of the small proportion of hypertensive persons under care and on medication are being inadequately treated, as judged by the effects of their treatment on blood pressure as compared with the optimal effects that are attainable with proper use of modern drugs.

Table 1-7. Death and Major Nonfatal Events in Untreated and Treated Hypertensives, Veterans Administration Cooperative Study Group on Antihypertensive Agents[a]

	Initial Diastolic Pressure			
	115–129 mm Hg		90–114 mm Hg	
	70 Untreated Men	73 Actively Treated Men	194 Untreated Men	186 Actively Treated Men
Cardiovascular deaths	4	0	19	8
Major nonfatal events[b]	23	2	57	14

[a] Average period of observation: Men with diastolic pressures of 115–129 mm Hg, 18 months; men with diastolic pressures of 90–114 mm Hg, 40 months.

[b] Includes congestive heart failure, cerebrovascular thrombosis, cerebral hemorrhage, myocardial infarction, grade 3 or 4 retinopathy, azotemia, severely elevated blood pressure.

From Freis et al. *J. A. M. A.*, Dec. 11, 1967, Vol. 202, p. 1028; Aug. 17, 1970, Vol. 213, p. 1143. Copyright 1967, 1970 American Medical Association.

Table 1-8. Effectiveness of Antihypertensive Treatment in Reducing Death and Major Nonfatal Events (Veterans Administration Cooperative Study Group on Antihypertensive Agents)

Initial Diastolic Blood Pressure	Deaths and Nonfatal Events (%)		Effectiveness of Treatment (%)[a]
	Control	Treated	
90–114	39.2	11.8	70
115–129	38.6	2.7	93

[a] Effectiveness of treatment is the difference between percents of incidence of events in control and treated groups, divided by percent incidence in control group.

From Freis et al. *J. A. M. A.*, Dec. 11, 1967, Vol. 202, p. 1028; Aug. 17, 1970, Vol. 213, p. 1143. Copyright 1967, 1970 American Medical Association.

Tables 1-7 and 1-8 and Figure 1-7 from the Veterans Administration study [13, 14] illustrate what good therapy can do in terms of morbidity and mortality. The data in Tables 1-7 and 1-8 dramatically demonstrate the efficacy of active therapy for men with severe hypertension (average baseline diastolic pressures 115–129 mm Hg): 2 morbid events in those treated versus 27 morbid events in those not treated. Therapy was 93 percent effective in preventing such events. With this highly significant positive result, it was ethically necessary to give active medication to the group on placebo. Thus, the trial was properly stopped after about 18 months, which was long before the originally planned five years.

For men with baseline diastolic pressures averaging 90–114 mm Hg, which is the most common range of diastolic pressures in hypertension, a significant positive result also was recorded. Of the 186 men randomly assigned to active treatment with a three-drug combination, morbid events developed in only 22, compared with 76 in the 194 men receiving placebo. Thus, in this group the risk that a morbid event would develop over five years was reduced from about 55 to 18 percent by treatment; that is, treatment was 67 percent effective in preventing complications. Death occurred in only 9 patients in the treated group but in 35 in the control group; 8 deaths related to hypertension or atherosclerosis occurred in the treated group and 19 in the control group. In addition, persistent elevation

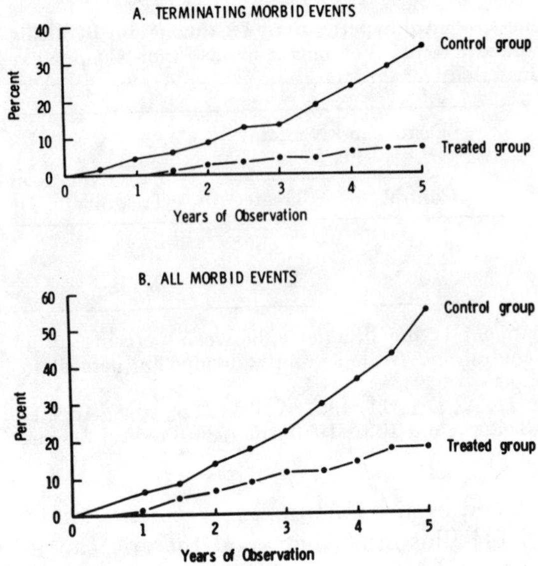

FIG. 1-7. Veterans Administration Cooperative Study on Antihypertensive Agents. Estimated cumulative incidence of morbidity over a five-year period in men with average diastolic blood pressures 90–114 mm Hg at beginning of study (calculated by life table method). (From Freis et al. *J.A.M.A.*, Aug. 17, 1970, Vol. 213, p. 1143. Copyright 1970 American Medical Association.)

of diastolic blood pressure to 125 mm Hg or more developed in 20 patients, all of whom were in the control group. The beneficial effect of treatment was more evident in the patients with higher initial blood pressures than in those with lower levels at entry into the study.

Treatment apparently was most effective in the prevention of congestive heart failure and stroke, less effective in preventing clinical manifestations of severe coronary atherosclerosis. The limited size of the study precluded a definitive assessment of the effectiveness in preventing premature coronary heart disease (CHD) by drug treatment of hypertension. However, the data currently available support the judgment that effective long-term therapy for hypertension may help to prevent CHD and other atherosclerotic diseases.

As a result of this research, the efficacy of treatment of hypertension is now much less in question than it was a few years ago, when some people could still say, "Maybe you do harm by lowering blood pressure, possibly by reducing coronary and cerebral perfusion, and therefore you'd better be careful." Now it is possible to be definitive about the value of therapy, at least for a much broader spectrum of hypertensive patients than heretofore. However, more data are needed on the effect of treatment in the mildest cases and in women. Particularly needed are data on the efficacy of treatment in reducing the risk of coronary disease in such persons—a key challenge strategically in terms of the role of hypertension as one of the three major risk factors contributing to the present-day epidemic of heart attacks [15]. More information is also needed on benefit-to-risk ratios for treatment that is continued for decades. For example, are there serious consequences over many years from "mild" thiazide-induced hyperglycemia, hyperuricemia, and hypokalemia? Experience is also needed in order to be able to generalize the positive Veterans Administration study experience in mass public health and medical practice. A major effort sponsored by the National Heart and Lung Institute is presently underway to clarify some of these questions (the Hypertension Detection and Follow-up Program).

Present Inadequacy of Hypertensive Management

A huge problem exists in this country in regard to inadequacy of care for hypertensive patients. A recent report of the Inter-Society Commission for Heart Disease Resources [16], gives data from three studies in the 1960s. Of all persons with hypertension in these community surveys, about 40 percent were unaware of their condition. About a third were under treatment, about half of whom were under control. Thus, no more than 20 percent of those with hypertension were receiving effective treatment.

More recent data are available from the Chicago Heart Association. These data were collected on almost 40,000 employed Chicagoans from November, 1967, through May, 1972 [17]. Table 1-9 presents data on the percentage of those with previously undetected hypertension in this screened population, aged 25–64 [17a]. Hypertension was defined using World

Table 1-9. Undetected, Untreated or Uncontrolled Hypertension in the Employed Population, Screenees age 25–64, Chicago Heart Association Detection Project in Industry, 1967–1972

Diagnostic and Therapeutic Status	White Males	Black Males	White Females	Black Fe-males
Not previously diagnosed but elevated at screening	61.9%	64.6%	48.3%	42.0%
Previously diagnosed, no current treatment, elevated at screening	18.1%	17.7%	18.1%	19.6%
On current treatment, but pressure elevated at screening	11.8%	11.3%	16.1%	17.4%
Undiagnosed, untreated, or uncontrolled (sum of rows 1–3)	91.8%	93.6%	82.5%	79.0%
On current treatment, normal screening pressure	8.2%	6.4%	17.5%	21.0%
Number of hypertensives[a]	3,560	283	2,027	219
All screenees	16,326	1,091	10,408	1,328

[a] Elevated blood pressure at screening (SBP ≧ 160 and/or DBP ≧ 95 mm Hg), or positive history of hypertension with current treatment and BP at screening not elevated.
From Stamler et al. [17a].

Health Organization criteria ($\geqq$ 160 mm Hg systolic and/or $\geqq$ 95 mm Hg diastolic for a single reading of casual blood pressure). The situation was no better—to put it conservatively—than in the early and mid-1960s. A majority of those with hypertension were unaware of their condition (row 1, Table 1-9); these are not the unemployed, not the victims of ghetto deprivation, but are gainfully employed persons. That is the first problem: a large number of cases of undetected hypertension.

The second problem, which is exemplified by rows 2 and 3 of Table 1-9, is the treatment problem. Of the screenees who already knew that they were hypertensive, a sizable proportion were not on treatment. Overall, therefore, only a minority of hypertensive persons were being treated.

More detailed analysis revealed that this was true for all educational levels and for white and black people alike. And it was true throughout the years 1967–1972. Apparently, publication of the two reports of the Veterans Administration studies on efficacy of treatment in the *Journal of the American Medical Association* in 1967 and 1970 [13, 14], which were reprinted extensively for physicians, had no impact in terms of increasing the percentage of hypertensive persons on treatment. If anything, that percentage declined from 1967 to 1972. Throughout this period it was even lower for persons aged 25–44 than for those 45–64, even though elevated blood pressure early in adulthood is especially likely to exert a harmful influence.

The findings with respect to effectiveness of therapy, for those on treatment when screened, again are cause for concern: Only half of those with hypertension who were on treatment had blood pressures below World Health Organization criteria for abnormal levels (rows 3 and 5, Table 1-9). This was true for men and women, white and black, both at ages 25–44 and 45–64. Thus, this study reveals no real evidence of improvement in the 1970s over the late 1960s.

A few studies have gone a step further and inquired as to the regularity of treatment. Clearly, if therapy is to be useful in preventing complications, it must be continued in effective form without interruption for years. Unfortunately, this, too,

Table 1-10. Survey of Treatment Status for Hypertension, Summer 1969, Middle-aged Hypertensive Men (Peoples Gas Company Study)

Group	Percent
All hypertensives	100.0
Aware of hypertension	93.9
History of treatment	66.5
History of regular treatment	29.9
On treatment now	39.0
DBP Reduced ≧ 6 mm Hg	11.6
DBP Reduced ≧ 16 mm Hg	4.3

From Stamler [4].

is rarely the case. Table 1-10 presents data from our study in the Peoples Gas Company in Chicago [4] of men who had been followed year after year by periodic physical examinations, were told that they had hypertension, and were referred to their private physicians. After about a decade of such follow-up, they were called in, interviewed about their treatment status, and examined briefly.

Amazingly enough, 6.1 percent professed not to know they were hypertensive. This is hard to believe, since they were repeatedly informed of their hypertensive status year after year. This is an example of the residual problems of communication. One-third were never treated, despite referrals year after year to their private physicians by the company medical department. The history of regular treatment was low; less than half received such treatment.

For those on treatment at the time of the survey, in less than one-third was the blood pressure reduced 6 mm Hg or more (based on the accumulated records of past years in the medical department charts), and in only one-tenth was there a reduction of 16 mm Hg or more. (Keep in mind that a fall of 16 mm Hg was the average residual reduction in the Veterans Administration study with baseline pressures in the range of 90–114 mm Hg.)

A simple set of figures—rough but reasonable approximations of the situation as revealed by the several population surveys—is very useful for boiling down the problem to its somber, harsh realities and pinpointing the challenge to our health education and medical care delivery system: ½ × ½ × ½. This means that in one-half of those with hypertension, it has previously been undetected; one-half those known to have hypertension are untreated; and one-half of those treated are inadequately treated. Therefore, in only one-eighth of the 20 to 25 million people with hypertension is the condition detected and adequately treated, based on the modest criterion of a current lowering of blood pressure to less than 160 mm Hg systolic and/or less than 95 mm Hg diastolic. For an optimal blood pressure response, lower values must be sustained over the long term. Conservatively, then, seven-eighths of those with hypertension—seven-eighths of 20 to 25 million persons—are being inadequately served.

Why Have We Failed?

Failure in Medical Practice

Why is this practice experience so unsatisfactory? Little has been done to clarify this problem, and it needs to be dealt with. Almost certainly, the heritage of therapeutic nihilism in regard to hypertension is part of the problem. Certain pieces of available information offer food for thought, for example, the data in Table 1-11. These findings indicate that for the person in whom hypertension has been diagnosed, lack of effective control *does not relate* to frequency of visits to physicians. The majority of the hypertensive men in the Peoples Gas Company were going to their physicians at least quarterly [4].

Patients often stop taking medication. In Baldwin County, Georgia, patients were asked, "Why did you stop taking medication?" As is evident in Table 1-12, financial considerations were one reason but not the main one [18]. They "didn't realize" they should continue; they "felt better"; they took drugs "when needed." Obviously, in this instance, successful doctor-patient communication on the importance of regular,

Table 1-11. Frequency of Visits to Physicians, 64 (of 164) Middle-aged Hypertensive Men Currently on Treatment, Survey of Treatment Status, Summer, 1969 (Peoples Gas Company Study)

Group	Percent	Cumulative Percent
All hypertensive patients currently on treatment	100.0	100.0
At least monthly visits to M.D.	32.8	32.8
At least quarterly visits to M.D.	23.4	56.2
At least semi-annual visits to M.D.	28.1	84.3
Annual or less frequent visits to M.D.	15.6	99.9

From Stamler [4].

Table 1-12. Reasons Why Treatment for Hypertension Was Discontinued (Baldwin County Hypertension Survey, 1962)

Number giving reasons	104
Total[a]	110%
Financial considerations	16%
Didn't realize should continue	12%
Felt better	30%
Take when needed	16%
Miscellaneous	36%

[a] Total is more than 100% because some gave more than one reason.
From Wilber, J. A. In Stamler, J., Stamler, R., and Pullman, T. N. (Eds.), *The Epidemiology of Hypertension,* Grune & Stratton, New York, 1967. By permission.

sustained, long-term therapy for hypertension had not been established. Chapter 5 deals with this type of problem in more detail.

When the nature of therapy is evaluated, it is clear that, by and large, the medical profession has not yet achieved high-level awareness of the potential for normalizing blood pressure with a high benefit-to-risk ratio through use of a *stepped care* approach to treatment, including combinations of medication when necessary, e.g., such triple combinations as were employed so effectively in the Veterans Administration study.

Only a minority of the patients on treatment in the Peoples Gas Company were taking such effective combinations at the time of our survey in 1969. Thus, dissemination of knowledge about optimal therapeutic regimen is obviously a big challenge in the area of physician education.

Figure 1-8 illustrates data collected in the Baldwin County study [18a]. At the time of the first mass survey in 1964, the treatment situation was deplorable. Therefore, a special pro-

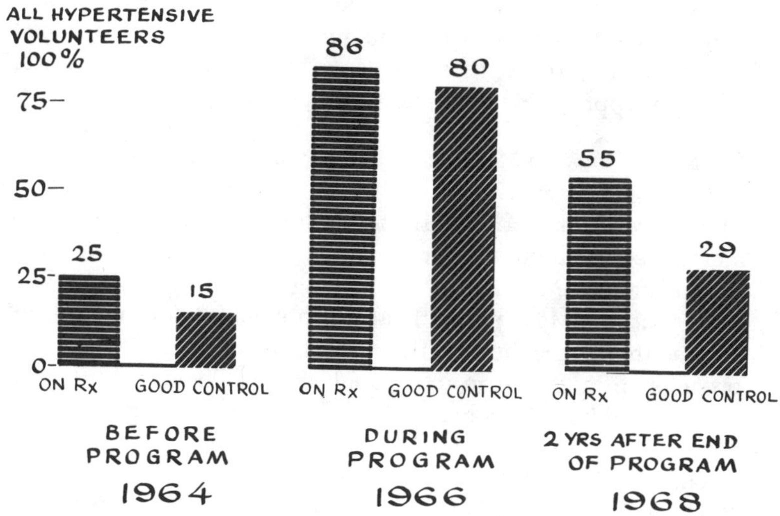

FIG. 1-8. Effects of home follow-up program on 88 hypertensive volunteers, Baldwin County, Georgia. Percentage of volunteers on treatment and with good blood pressure control before, during, and two years after program. (Adapted from Wilber and Barrow [18a].)

gram was begun to try to improve prescription and adherence. A home visiting program by nurses was instituted. Good control was defined as diastolic pressure under 95 mm Hg. The rates went up to 86 percent on treatment and 80 percent under good control. Clearly, this program showed that it is possible to improve therapeutic status for a majority of patients with hypertension. In Chapter 5, Dr. Moser comments on the applicability of this type of study to private practice.

The pilot program in Baldwin County was discontinued, having proved its efficacy! Not unexpectedly, when the firm, steady persuasion and education characteristic of such a program stopped, things changed markedly: Two years after the end of the program, both treatment status and effectiveness of control had regressed (Fig. 1-8).

The lesson from this and other experiences [19] is clear: In any medical care program for chronic disease, good long-term sustained therapy can and must be systematically assured by a combination of efforts involving both individual health professionals working with individual patients and supplementary resources generated and organized by the community. This is necessary for sustained success, not only to control hypertension by modern pharmacologic means, but also to achieve long-term adherence to such goals as cessation of cigarette smoking, appropriate diet, and weight control.

Failure to Develop Mass Programs for the Control of Hypertension

The entire history of modern public health teaches this fundamental lesson about the control of mass disease problems—a lesson highly relevant to the challenge of effective control of hypertension: Mass public health problems require mass public health approaches to their solution, i.e., community approaches in addition to individual efforts. The simple doctor-patient relationship is not by itself capable of doing the entire job.

This fundamental point was made over a decade ago, in 1964, at the Second National Conference on Cardiovascular Diseases, cosponsored by the American Heart Association, the Heart Disease Control Program of the Public Health Service, and the National Heart Institute. Some of the recommendations in its Community Service Summary Report are as follows:

Hypertension as defined by the World Health Organization is a problem which is amenable to community efforts in detection, and management.

Case finding is essential but of little value unless it is followed by referral to sources of medical care and systematic follow-up.

Physicians should be shown the importance of early and adequate treatment of mild benign hypertension. . . .

In 1974, the Inter-Society Commission for Heart Disease Resources [7] reaffirmed this basic concept and elaborated specific approaches for its implementation and fulfillment. While this report merits complete reading and detailed study, mention of particularly salient portions is useful here. (The sections that deal with early detection, methods of follow-up, and resources will be found in the Appendix to this chapter.)

The Commission recommended the commitment of money and manpower to reach the following goals: (1) *the prevention or control of hyperlipidemia, obesity, hypertension, and diabetes by changes in diet;* (2) *the elimination of cigarette smoking;* (3) *the control of elevated blood pressure by the use of pharmacologic agents.* The Commission called for a major national effort to detect and control hypertension and to establish and expand community programs designed to detect and treat all persons, regardless of age, who, because of a combination of major risk factors, are very susceptible to premature atherosclerotic diseases. It also recommended community programs to assist hypertensive patients in obtaining long-term treatment:

On the basis of recent experience, detection programs are likely to identify a very large proportion of the population, e.g., about 20 or 30 percent of middle-aged adults, as being at unusually high risk. For such individuals, community services should be provided to assist their physicians in long-term management. Such programs will require the training and use of large numbers of allied health personnel, as well as physicians [16].

The Commission emphasized that in the long run it should be cheaper to control hypertension than "to care for those who become disabled and economically unproductive as a consequence of the disease." A community hypertension control program will be successful, the Commission stated, only if it develops "techniques for continued physician and patient education, effective longitudinal patient follow-up and care, and means to provide free or low-cost drugs. . . ." The Commission also suggested that case detection for hypertension can easily be made a part of most multiphasic screening programs and that it is necessary to convince community planners that major health and economic benefits for large numbers of people in our society will result from control of hypertension [16].

Economic Aspects of Hypertension

Projected Costs

If the Commission's points are valid, the effort to control hypertension, like other preventive efforts to control mass diseases, such as cholera, smallpox, typhoid, pellagra, scurvy, and rickets, should more than pay for itself financially. Some data are available that permit a preliminary assessment of economic cost of hypertension. The American Heart Association has published projections of costs of cardiovascular diseases for 1973 [11] (Figure 1-9), and the 1971 Report of the

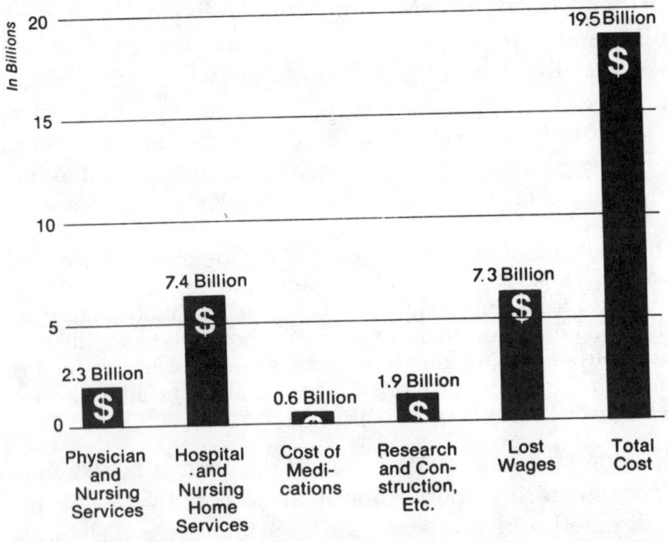

FIG. 1-9. Estimated economic costs of cardiovascular diseases by type of expenditure, United States, 1973. (From American Heart Association [11], © 1972, American Heart Association, Inc., reprinted with permission.

National Heart and Lung Institute Task Force on Arteriosclerosis [20] gives the most detailed estimate for 1967, including estimates specifically of the costs of hypertension per se (Table 1-13).

Morbidity, disability, and mortality from hypertensive disease alone among people under age 65 in the productive years of life has been costing the nation over 1 billion dollars annually in indirect costs. Since hypertension is a major risk factor, contributing significantly to at least one-third of the heart attacks and strokes, roughly another 3.5 billion dollars in indirect costs of hypertensive disease prior to age 65 lie concealed in these categories, adding up to about 4.5 billion dollars in indirect costs. A similar calculation gives a direct cost estimate, irrespective of age, of almost 2 billion dollars. It is reasonable to estimate that at least one-quarter of this money, i.e., about half a billion dollars, was spent for persons under age 65. Therefore, the total cost of hypertensive disease among

Table 1-13. Estimated Economic Costs to the Nation Due to Morbidity and Mortality from Arteriosclerotic and Hypertensive Diseases, United States, 1967

	Amount (in millions)			
		Morbidity		
Diagnosis	Total	Direct Costs	Indirect Costs	Mortality Costs[a]
Total (arteriosclerotic or hypertensive)	$23,887	$4,291	$1,133	$18,463
Arteriosclerotic heart disease	15,545	2,072	370	13,103
Stroke[b]	4,605	971	235	3,399
Diseases of arteries	1,082	354	31	697
Hypertensive diseases[c]	2,655	894	497	1,264

[a] Present value of lifetime earnings (discounted at 6%) of persons who died of arteriosclerotic and hypertensive diseases.
[b] Includes 20% not due to arteriosclerosis.
[c] Does not include all arteriosclerotic disease in which hypertension was involved.
From Task Force on Arteriosclerosis of the National Heart and Lung Institute [20].

persons under age 65 was about 5 billion dollars for 1967. For all ages, the total cost was over 9 billion. And that was seven years ago. Given the general inflationary trend since, and the even steeper rise in the costs of medical care, it is reasonable to estimate that hypertensive disease will cost this nation about 15 billion dollars in 1974.

Evidence That Disease Can Be Reduced

The data of the Veterans Administration field trials indicate that effective comprehensive control programs can cut disease by over 50 percent. It therefore seems reasonable to project a well-planned program for the coming years and to provide an adequate budget for its accomplishment. We are currently spending hundreds of millions of dollars for renal dialysis programs. It seems logical to expend equal amounts in an effort to *prevent* renal disease, as well as cerebrovascular and cardiac disease, and to budget for this purpose amounts that can really begin to accomplish something. As yet, only a minimal effort has been mounted.

One positive development has taken place at the federal level: The National High Blood Pressure Education Program has begun. However, only a penny per American, or 10 cents per hypertensive person, has thus far been allocated to the Department of Health, Education, and Welfare to carry out this professional and public education campaign. Nor will education alone be enough. Public health experience teaches that education programs without closely linked control programs, that is, programs to facilitate action, based on the knowledge acquired, do not accomplish much. This is especially likely to be true for a disease like hypertension, which may be present for years without symptoms and millions of whose victims have low incomes and are black, with restricted access to needed long-term care. Federal leadership and resources are needed for the step-by-step building of a national program.

Some Approaches to the Possible Primary Prevention of Hypertensive Disease

The development of an effective national program to identify, evaluate, and treat 20 million or more hypertensive persons in the United States is certainly a huge and complex task, requiring a great deal of careful hard work. But that challenge should not blind us to a basic fact: in the long run, the ultimate solution of the hypertension problem is primary prevention, not case finding and drug treatment, important as they are now. Of course, solution of the riddle of the etiopathogenesis of essential hypertension will certainly add strength to a primary prevention effort. Thus, every encouragement must be given to continuation and expansion of the basic research assault at every level. But does present knowledge already provide a foundation for a rational and safe approach to the primary prevention of hypertension, that is, for the prevention of essential hypertension?

Control of Salt Intake

Sound "handles" exist now that can and should be grasped in an effort at primary prevention. First, there is the considerable body of evidence from experimental, epidemiologic, and clinicopharmacologic studies implicating dietary salt in the etiopathogenesis of essential hypertension. The evidence has been considerable for years, and it keeps mounting, that habitual high salt intake acts as a "conditioner," setting the stage for elevated blood pressure, at least in genetically susceptible animals and human beings [15, 21, 22]. Certainly, it makes good sense to develop a sustained effort to encourage the American people to eat less salt and to encourage the food industry to reduce the salt in their products. This long-term undertaking in the general population, in the best traditions of successful public health practice, should involve the development of ways to focus especially on hypertension-prone families.

Control of Obesity

Extensive evidence demonstrates unequivocally that overweight in youth, young adulthood, and middle age and gains in weight in the years from young adulthood into middle age are associated with an increase in risk of hypertension [15, 21]. Figures 1-10 and 1-11 provide some of this evidence. In Figure 1-10, from the Peoples Gas Company study [15], relative weight is based on the Framingham standard. The three groups are the "not obese or only slightly obese," "mod-

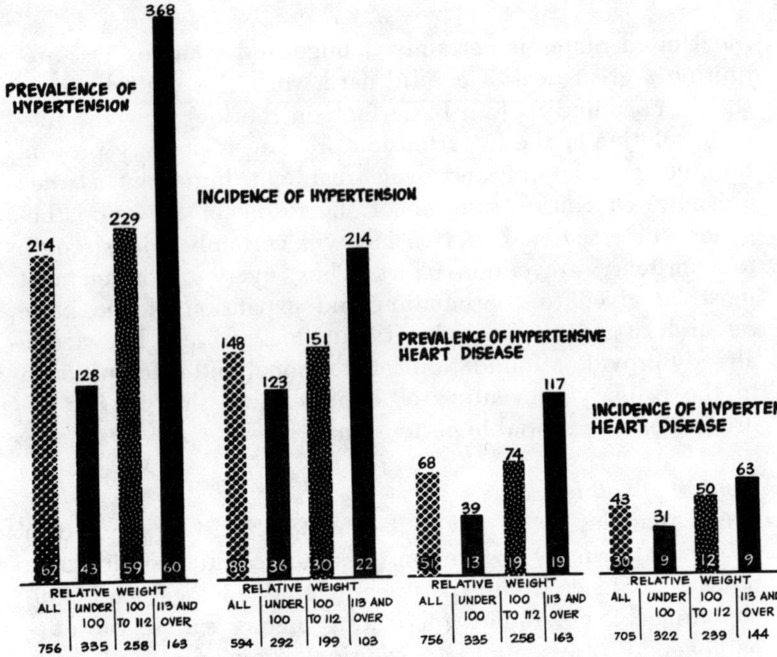

FIG. 1-10. Relationship between relative weight and prevalence and incidence of hypertension and hypertensive heart disease (756 men originally aged 50–59 on January 1, 1954) with follow-up through December 31, 1957. (From Stamler, J. *Lectures on Preventive Cardiology*. Grune & Stratton, New York, 1967. By permission.)

erately obese," and "markedly obese." Illustrated are the prevalence of hypertension per thousand at first examination and the subsequent development of new hypertension over the next four years. The prevalence of hypertensive heart disease at first examination and the incidence of new hypertensive heart disease over the next four years are also shown [15].

Figure 1-11 presents data from an analysis that is more sophisticated in one respect, i.e., it not only shows relative weight at one time (in this case, in young adulthood), but also slight, moderate, or marked weight gain over the next 20 or more years. The higher the relative weight initially, the greater the tendency to elevated blood pressure in middle age, and, both for those lean in youth and overweight in youth, the greater the gain in weight from young adulthood to middle age, the greater the tendency to high blood pressure.

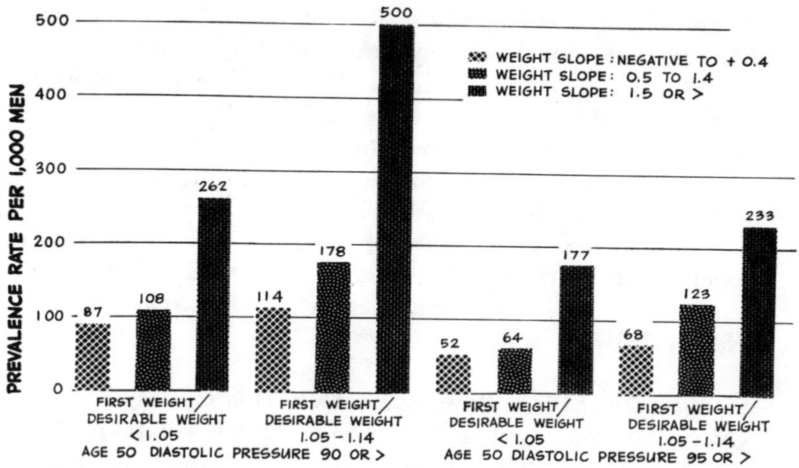

FIG. 1-11. Relationship between initial weight ratio as a young adult, slope of the weight curve over the next 20 years, and development of hypertensive disease in those years (follow-up data on 746 men aged 40–59 in 1958–1959). (From Stamler, J. *Lectures on Preventive Cardiology*. Grune & Stratton, New York, 1967. By permission.)

Every analysis of this relationship has yielded similar sets of data from many parts of the world [23]. However, hypertension does not develop in every obese person nor in every weight gainer. Almost certainly, besides simple avoirdupois, other factors are at work, possibly including aspects of sodium metabolism; and, once again, genetic susceptibility probably enters in. But whatever the mechanism, it is a reasonable inference that effective mass public health efforts to improve American nutritional and exercise habits and thereby prevent and control obesity, including the now all-too-common obesity among young people, might be useful for the primary prevention of a significant proportion of our hypertensive disease problem.

There are also some data demonstrating that when obese people reduce, on the average they experience a reduction in blood pressure [23]. Here again, a broad, sustained, population-wide effort needs to be accompanied by special measures pinpointed at those susceptible to hypertension, i.e., already obese children, young adults, and middle-aged persons and members of families with a history of hypertension.

Importance of Family History of Hypertension

The Peoples Gas Company study [15] illustrates the importance of a positive family history of hypertension in identifying those possibly susceptible to hypertension. The comparative incidence of hypertension, particularly of frankly elevated blood pressure (diastolic 100 mm Hg or more) in populations stratified by either a negative or positive family history, yields clear evidence of a familial tendency. If both parents are involved, the risks are especially great. This tendency can be shown as early as the first or second decade of life [24, 25].

Significance of Blood Pressure Levels in Youth

Overweight and family history are not the sole criteria for finding those susceptible to hypertension. From young adulthood on, blood pressure itself, within the generally accepted range of normotension, is an important predictor. The research evidence on this is now sizable, although, regrettably, its practical implications have not yet been grasped either by medical or public health practitioners. It has been found that young and middle-aged persons with high normal levels for their age and sex tend to have a steeper slope of blood pressure increase over the next years and decades than those with low and medium normal pressures [26, 27].

Similarly, there is no doubt that "spiked" patterns of blood pressure levels early in life are prognostically significant. This is shown in Figure 1-12, in which data from chart records on employees of the Peoples Gas Company in Chicago [15] are presented. The data consist of a single blood pressure value for each man employed 20 or more years: the blood pressure obtained when he first began to work for the company as a youth or young adult. This set of data deals with the question: How does such a blood pressure in young adulthood relate to the risk of elevation in middle age (20 or more years later) and to the risk of having a clinical diagnosis of hypertension or hypertensive heart disease? Clearly, those who showed "spiked" patterns of blood pressure in youth are at greater risk in later years.

Similar data are available from the home office of the Metropolitan Life Insurance Company, where the blood

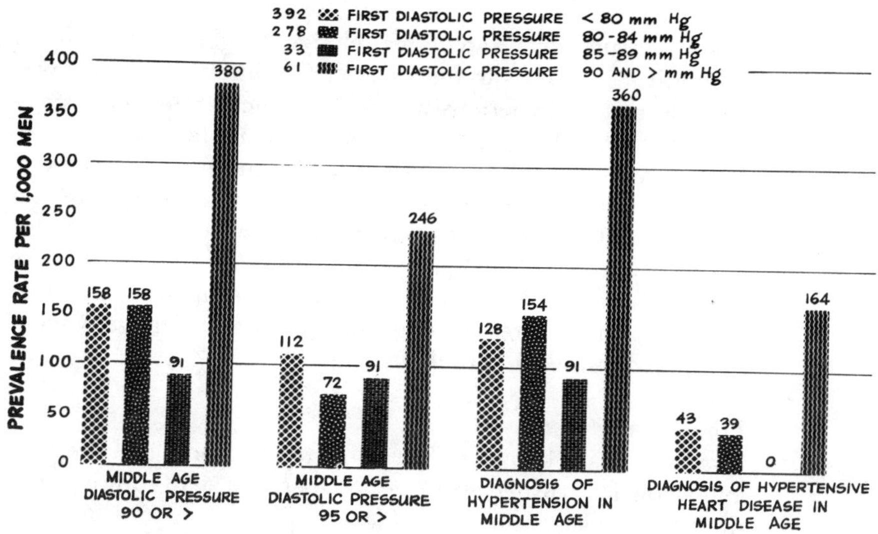

FIG. 1-12. Relationship between initial blood pressure reading as a young adult and subsequent development of hypertensive disease in middle age (20-year follow-up data on 746 men aged 40–59 in 1958–1959). (From Stamler, J. *Lectures on Preventive Cardiology*. Grune & Stratton, New York, 1967. By permission.)

pressures of the staff have been followed for years, and from studies of United States Army Officers. The data of Paffenbarger et al. [8, 27] on college entrants have similar implications. The "spiked" blood pressure patterns of teen-agers and young adults in high school or college and in preemployment or Armed Forces physical examinations are not to be ignored, because they are significant in terms of future disease.

Heart Rate and Risk of Hypertension

From both the older and the more recent literature, another trait associated with increased risk of developing hypertension is rapid resting heart rate, that is, a rate in the 80s, 90s, or more per minute. Studies of Army officers, Harvard and University of Pennsylvania graduates, and Chicago population groups have all demonstrated this relationship [15, 27].

Glucose Intolerance and Hyperuricemia

Recent data from our group indicate that glucose intolerance and hyperuricemia are independently and additively related to blood pressure, over and above relative weight and heart rate. When these several variables were used simultaneously, it was possible to find hypertensive persons concentrated in a small proportion of the population with a combination of overweight, rapid heart rate, hyperglycemia, and hyperuricemia. It remains to be seen from prospective analyses whether or not glucose intolerance and hyperuricemia are as truly predictive of the future development of hypertension as are positive family history, high normal levels of blood pressure, transient "spikes" of blood pressure into the hypertensive range, weight gain and obesity, and rapid heart rate.

Preventive Measures

The list of traits known to be related to elevated blood pressure and known or suspected to be independent and additive predictors of hypertension is sizable:

1. Positive family history.
2. High normal blood pressure in youth, young adulthood, or middle age.
3. "Spikes" of blood pressure into the hypertensive range in youth or young adulthood.
4. Overweight.
5. Rapid heart rate.
6. Possibly glucose intolerance.
7. Possibly hyperuricemia.

How does knowledge of these predictors provide approaches to the primary prevention of hypertension? First of all it offers means for the early identification of susceptible persons. Years of epidemiologic and public health experience indicate that such identification is always useful for developing preventive programs, since it gives a focus for action. What action should be taken for the primary prevention of hypertension? The following nutritional-hygienic measures are rational in terms of our present knowledge and may be useful:

1. Consumption of a habitual diet that has a moderate, not high, salt content.
2. Avoidance or correction of obesity through proper nutrition

and exercise. (This may also aid in control of glucose intolerance and perhaps even of hyperuricemia.)

3. Regular frequent exercise of the rhythmic type from youth on (e.g., vigorous walking, biking, swimming), not only to maintain proper body weight, but also to achieve cardiopulmonary fitness, with consequent slowing of heart rate and parasympathetic "dominance."
4. Moderation in intake of saturated fat and cholesterol (as well as of calories and salt) and avoidance of cigarettes. These are adjuvant measures to assure the broadest possible nutritional-hygienic program for minimizing the risk of adult cardiovascular disease generally.

While no proof is available that these measures will indeed achieve the primary prevention of hypertension or its complications, they are reasonable inferences from available data, and they are safe.

But if this program is sensible and reasonable, it also has many practical implications in terms of implementation. First of all, it means targeting hypertension-prone people, ideally early in life, by mass public health work, in practicing physicians' offices, in efforts by health departments, schools, factories, insurance companies, and the military. And for such persons, sound programs are needed to advise and guide them on safe nutritional-hygienic approaches to primary prevention—programs linked to their sources of medical care. In addition to such nutritional-hygienic advice, such persons should be kept under long-term medical surveillance, with the good reasons for this made clear to them in ways calculated to prevent negative psychological effects. This is necessary not only for proper evaluation of this new endeavor, but also to permit early institution of pharmacologic treatment if, despite the effort, blood pressure rises into the frankly hypertensive range.

This kind of challenge and the related matters of public education, professional education, and development of new services need concerted long-term attention. It is time now to launch at least pilot programs on the primary prevention of high blood pressure. A beginning can, and should, be made today to meet this greatest challenge of all in the hypertension field.

Acknowledgments

It is a pleasure to acknowledge the cooperation of the author's senior colleagues in the long-term investigations presented here; especially Howard Adler, Ph.D., David M. Berkson, M.D., Alan Dyer, Ph.D., Morton B. Epstein, Ph.D., Yolanda Hall, M.S., Howard A. Lindberg, M.D., Louise Mojonnier, Ph.D., James A. Schoenberger, M.D., Richard Shekelle, Ph.D., and Rose Stamler, M.A.

Appreciation is also expressed to the following colleagues and publishers for permission to cite from published works: Nemat Borhani, M.D., Edward Lew, Ph.D., Edward D. Freis, M.D., Dean Krueger, Iwao Moriyama, M.D., Ralph S. Paffenbarger, M.D., Joseph A. Wilber, M.D., The American Heart Association, *American Journal of Public Health,* Grune & Stratton, Harvard University Press, *Journal of the American Medical Association, Minnesota Medicine.*

The author's research has been supported by the American Heart Association, Chicago Heart Association, Illinois Regional Medical Program, and the National Heart and Lung Institute, National Institutes of Health, United States Public Health Service.

References

1. U.S. Department of Health, Education, and Welfare. *Blood Pressure of Adults by Race and Area, United States, 1960–1962.* National Health Examination Survey, National Center for Health Statistics, Series 11, Number 5, 1964.
2. U.S. Department of Health, Education, and Welfare. *Hypertension and Hypertensive Heart Disease in Adults, United States, 1960–1962.* National Health Examination Survey, National Center for Health Statistics, Series 11, Number 13, 1966.
3. Wilber, J. A., and Barrow, J. G. Hypertension—A community problem. *Am. J. Med.* 52:653, 1972.
4. Stamler, J. High Blood Pressure in the United States—An Overview of the Problem and the Challenge. *National Conference on High Blood Pressure Education—Report of Proceedings.* U.S. Department of Health, Education, and Welfare, Public Health Service, National Institutes of Health, DHEW Publication No. (NIH) 73-486, 1973. P. 11.
5. Schoenberger, J. A., et al. Current status of hypertension control in an industrial population. *J. A. M. A.* 222:559, 1972.
6. Lew, E. A. Blood Pressure and Mortality—Life Insurance Experience. In Stamler, J., Stamler, R., and Pullman, T. N. (Eds.), *The Epidemiology of Hypertension.* Grune & Stratton, New York, 1967. P. 392.
7. Inter-Society Commission for Heart Disease Resources. Atherosclerosis Study Group and Epidemiology Study Group. Pri-

mary Prevention of the Atherosclerotic Diseases. In Wright, I. S. and Fredrickson, D. T. (Eds.), *Cardiovascular Diseases—Guidelines for Prevention and Care,* U.S. Government Printing Office, Washington, D.C., 1974. P. 15.

8. Paffenbarger, R. S., et al. Chronic disease in former college students. II. Methods of study and observations on mortality from coronary heart disease. *Am. J. Public Health* 56:962, 1966.
9. Stamler, J., Berkson, D. M., and Lindberg, H. A. Risk Factors: Their Role in the Etiology and Pathogenesis of the Atherosclerotic Diseases. In Wissler, R. W., and Geer, J. C. (Eds.), *Pathogenesis of Atherosclerosis.* Williams & Wilkins, Baltimore, 1972. P. 41.
10. Lerner, P. R. *Social Security Disability Applicant Statistics, 1969.* U.S. Department of Health, Education, and Welfare, Social Security Administration, Office of Research and Statistics, DHEW Publication Number (SSA) 74-1911, U.S. Government Printing Office, Washington, D.C., 1973.
11. American Heart Association. *1973 Heart Facts,* EM 509A. New York, 1972.
12. Moriyama, I. M., Krueger, D. E., and Stamler, J. *Cardiovascular Diseases in the United States.* Harvard University Press, Cambridge, Mass., 1971.
13. Freis, E., et al. Veterans Administration Cooperative Study Group on Antihypertensive Agents. Effects of treatment on morbidity in hypertension. I. Results in patients with diastolic blood pressures averaging 115 through 129 mm Hg. *J.A.M.A.* 202:1028, 1967.
14. Freis, E., et al. Veterans Administration Cooperative Study Group on Antihypertensive Agents. Effects of treatment on morbidity in hypertension. II. Results in patients with diastolic blood pressure averaging 90 though 114 mm Hg. *J.A.M.A.* 213:1143, 1970.
15. Stamler, J. *Lectures on Preventive Cardiology.* Grune & Stratton, New York, 1967.
16. Inter-Society Commission for Heart Disease Resources. Hypertension Study Group. Guidelines for the Detection, Diagnosis, and Management of Hypertensive Populations. In Wright, I. S., and Fredrickson, D. T. (Eds.), *Cardiovascular Diseases—Guidelines for Prevention and Care.* U.S. Government Printing Office, Washington, D.C., 1974. P. 186.
17. Stamler, J., et al. Hypertension: The Problem and the Challenge. *The Hypertension Handbook.* Merck, Sharp & Dohme, West Point, Pa., 1974. P.3.

17a. Stamler, J., Stamler, R., and Curry, C. L. *Hypertension in the Inner City.* New York Media Company, Inc., New York, 1974.

18. Wilber, J. A. Detection and Control of Hypertensive Disease in Georgia, U.S.A. In Stamler, J., Stamler, R., and Pullman, T. N. (Eds.), *The Epidemiology of Hypertension.* Grune & Stratton, New York, 1967. P. 439.
18a. Wilber, J. A., and Barrow, J. G. Reducing elevated blood pressure—Experience found in a community. *Minn. Med.* 52:1303, 1969.
19. Finnerty, F. A., Jr., Mattie, E. C., and Finnerty, F. A., III. Hypertension in the inner city. Part I. Analysis of clinic dropouts. *Circulation* 47:73, 1973.
20. Task Force on Arteriosclerosis of the National Heart and Lung Institute. *Arteriosclerosis,* Vol. II. U.S. Department of Health, Education, and Welfare, Public Health Service, DHEW Publication Number (NIH) 72-219, Washington, D.C., June, 1971.
21. Stamler, J., Stamler, R., and Pullman, T. N. (Eds.). *The Epidemiology of Hypertension.* Grune & Stratton, New York, 1967.
22. Dahl, L. K. Salt and hypertension. *Am. J. Clin. Nutr.* 25:231, 1972.
23. Chiang, B. N., Perlman, L. V., and Epstein, F. H. Overweight and hypertension—A review. *Circulation* 39:403, 1969.
24. Kass, E. H., and Zinner, S. H. How early can the tendency toward hypertension be detected? *Milbank Mem. Fund Q.* 47:(No. 3, Part 2), 143, 1969.
25. Deutscher, S., Epstein, F. H., and Kjelsberg, M. O. Familial aggregation of factors associated with coronary heart disease. *Circulation* 33:911, 1966.
26. Miall, W. E., and Lovell, H. G. Relation between change of blood pressure and age. *Br. Med. J.* 2:660, 1967.
27. Paffenbarger, R. S., Thorne, M. C., and Wing, A. L. Chronic disease in former college students. VIII. Characteristics in youth predisposing to hypertension in later years. *Am. J. Epidemiol.* 88:25, 1968.

Appendix*

Early Detection

Hypertension is usually an asymptomatic disease in its early phases . . . It is unrealistic, therefore, to rely on symptoms alone to prompt patients to seek medical care. There are essentially two approaches to finding hypertensives in the population: incidental screening and organized community screening . . . for effective hypertension control, most communities must supplement incidental screening with organized community programs for recording blood pressure in asymptomatic persons. . . .

* From Inter-Society Commission for Heart Disease Resources [16].

The population between 15 and 65 years of age, especially the black population, should be routinely screened. To reach this goal, most communities will have to plan long-range programs and establish priorities.

Undetected and untreated hypertension is also quite common in any low income group—irrespective of geography or ethnic mix. Because of the high prevalence of all diseases and social ills in such disadvantaged areas, it is especially important that hypertension screening be incorporated as a part of comprehensive health maintenance programs for these populations. Unless adequate diagnostic and treatment resources are provided for all disorders found, screening of any kind will serve only as another source of mounting frustration.

Finally, the prognosis of hypertension in the age group 15–30 years is particularly poor and these individuals should be identified and treated as early as possible. . . .

It is extremely important that better use be made of the information regarding patients with hypertension identified by various types of incidental screening programs. This effort requires more comprehensive professional education concerning the necessity for following and treating these patients, and more effective patient education regarding the importance of early diagnosis and adequate long-term management. Various methods to assure maximum follow-up of those patients identified through incidental screening should be developed and evaluated in each community.

Hypertensives identified in community screening programs should be referred. Since there is a tendency for many patients to ignore screening findings, repeated follow-up is usually required, and intensive educational programs for patients and their families may be necessary to assure cooperation.

To be successful, any community program for the early recognition of hypertension must be accompanied by intensive professional and public education. Professionals should be alerted to the significance of hypertension as a serious disease and the importance of long-term follow-up for the labile hypertensive. They should be made aware of the recent evidence that therapy both decreases the rate of damage to the vascular system and prevents complications, and they should know that even patients with moderate hypertension may benefit from effective treatment. It should be emphasized that hypertension is not a curable disease in most instances and must be evaluated periodically for the duration of the patient's life. Hypertension carries a familial relationship, and its presence in one member of the family should alert physicians to screen relatives for unsuspected or untreated disease. If teenagers are screened, special instructions should be sent to physicians outlining the importance of borderline blood pressure levels and guidelines for therapy in this population. If the screening program is to succeed, it is essential that the professional education program precede that of the public. However, an intensive public information program will be necessary before and during the community screening. . . .

Resources for Therapy
Since two-thirds of the patients identified as hypertensive are either not aware of their disease or have discontinued therapy, screening programs may triple the case load requiring treatment. Long-range local planning will be required to manage effectively this patient population without seriously overloading existing medical facilities.

Existing medical services often fail to provide satisfactory long-term care for patients with hypertension as evidenced by the large number who either leave therapy or receive inadequate treatment. In particular, economically underprivileged urban residents require more individualized management than can presently be provided in the depersonalized and overcrowded outpatient clinics of many large municipal and community hospitals. The development and evaluation of new and more effective techniques for delivering long-term care to all hypertensive patients is urgently needed. The proposed stratified system for organizing community resources for hypertension control, incorporating the concept of the neighborhood hypertension unit, represents one possible solution. Since this approach is relatively new, initial testing in the form of pilot studies will be necessary to evaluate effectiveness and feasibility and to make necessary modifications to meet local needs. Implementation of the system and the neighborhood unit concept and tailoring it to meet local needs necessarily involves a long-range organized approach to community and regional planning. . . .

Comments

The two Inter-Society Commission Reports were originally published in 1970 and 1971, respectively. Only the barest beginning has been made in the implementation of their recommendations.

Essentially, it is still unclear whether these reports and their recommendations will indeed become effective guidelines of a determined national effort or—like the 1964 Report of the Second National Conference on Cardiovascular Diseases—will become neglected tomes doomed to gather dust in the archives and libraries.

It is therefore necessary to go beyond the biomedical and health aspects of the hypertension problem and to discuss the humanistic, social, medical, and financial aspects. The classic mission of medicine, to give mankind added years of better life, must continue to be regarded as the overriding determinant of public policy and national priority.

2. The Role of Sodium, Volume, and the Kidney in Hypertension

Louis Tobian

Interest in the relation between salt and hypertension originally centered on the lowering of hypertensive blood pressures with diets very low in sodium chloride. Many years ago, F. M. Allen vigorously urged low-salt diets. In 1944, Kempner [1] introduced the rice diet for hypertension, the antihypertensive effect resulting from the diet's low salt content. Even a week on a high salt intake would slightly raise the blood pressure of subjects with established hypertension. McQuarrie showed definitively that a high salt intake would produce hypertension in a 13-year-old boy and that a normal salt intake would bring the blood pressure back to normal.

Provocative animal experiments were also performed in these early days. Lenel, Katz, and Rodbard made chickens hypertensive by giving them only a 1% saline solution for drinking water, and Sapirstein achieved a similar effect in rats by allowing them to drink only a 2% saline solution. In the classic experiment of Meneely et al. [2], various diets were prepared containing salt in very small, very large, or various intermediate amounts. The diets were fed to rats over a nine-month period, and it was found that each increment in salt intake brought a concomitant increase in blood pressure. Severe hypertension developed in the rats eating a dry diet containing 10 percent salt. With 2–5 percent salt in the diet, borderline or mild hypertension was observed. At the higher levels of blood pressure, obvious nephrosclerosis was encountered. In these early days, it was also clear that the full expression of deoxycorticosterone (hormone-induced) hypertension in the rat could best be obtained if deoxycorticosterone-treated rats had a high sodium chloride intake.

Conversely, a very low sodium intake completely prevented a rise in blood pressure after deoxycorticosterone. Potassium ingestion reduced the hypertension resulting from concomitant high sodium feeding.

Population Studies of Salt Intake

Reports such as these prompted epidemiologic studies of the relation between salt intake and hypertension. Prior and Evans [3] noted that the natives in small villages in New Guinea had virtually no hypertension and that blood pressures in the old men were no higher than those in the young men, demonstrating that blood pressure does not necessarily rise with advancing age. Genetically similar natives nearly always manifested some hypertension when they moved to modern coastal cities, and the salt in the urban diet was suspected as a cause of this emergence of hypertension.

Page [4] recently extended these observations to Solomon Island natives. In one primitive inland village no hypertension at all was found, and there was no rise of average blood pressure with advancing age. However, in another primitive village located on an offshore island, a significant amount of hypertension was observed, and the average blood pressure tended to rise with advancing age. The main difference between these two villages was that the natives living by the ocean cooked their fish in sea water. Fish cooked in this manner has a salt content of about 3 percent. Thus, this population was provided with significantly more dietary sodium than the inland group received.

Shaper [5] reported that the salt intake of Samburu herdsmen increases their salt intake to 18 gm a day when they are drafted into the army and begin to eat army rations. This high salt intake has no effect on their blood pressure during the first year of service, but, starting with the second year, their blood pressure begins to rise.

Moser [6] found an extremely high incidence of hypertension and strokes in the Bahamas, where salt intake is considerably higher than in the United States.

Japanese farmers in the northern prefecture of Akita eat a huge amount of salt daily, since salt is used in the preservation of their food. They may eat as much as 20–35 gm of salt per day, as compared with an average intake of 10 gm per day in the United States. In 84 percent of the farm villagers in this area, the systolic blood pressure is over 140 mm Hg [7], and the leading cause of death is stroke.

To sum up these population studies: In areas where the population has a very high salt intake, the incidence of hypertension is high. Where the salt intake is low (less than 4 gm of sodium chloride daily), the incidence of hypertension is low, and blood pressure does not rise with advancing years. A salt intake as low as 4 gm daily is compatible with very vigorous health.

In the United States, Dahl [8] found that the employees of Brookhaven National Laboratory who did not salt their food had approximately a 1 percent incidence of hypertension, while 12.7 percent of those who salted their food heavily had hypertension. Although Gifford [9] could not find any relationship between salt intake and the incidence of hypertension in the Cleveland area, he did note that heavy salt users had significantly more complications from their hypertension than did the light users of salt.

Salt and Animal Hypertension

In rats, hypertension can be induced with high-sodium feedings, and the hypertension will persist indefinitely, even after a normal diet is resumed [10]. It is as if the salt and the hypertension have somehow produced a permanent change, especially in the kidney, so that hypertension becomes a permanent adaptation. The same mechanism may be involved in the permanent hypertension that occurs after deoxycorticosterone therapy.

Dahl et al. [11] advanced an intriguing concept with regard to salt intake and hypertension. Everyone knows people who eat huge amounts of salt but still have a normal blood pressure and live to a fine old age. It is certain that essential hypertension has a strong hereditary aspect, and those who are highly resistant to hypertension will not be affected by an average salt intake. To document the principle of such hereditary resistance and susceptibility, from a single strain of rats, Dahl et al. bred a race very susceptible to salt hypertension and a race highly resistant to it. The resistant rats were also relatively resistant to all other forms of experimental hypertension except one-kidney Goldblatt hypertension [11]. When these two strains of rats were fed a diet reasonably low in sodium (0.3 percent), their blood pressures were similar while young. However, in adulthood, the hypertension-prone strain had blood pressures about 15 mm Hg higher than those of the hypertension-resistant strain. Thus, a form of high-normal, or borderline, essential hypertension developed in sensitive rats eating a low-salt diet.

In my view, it is very reasonable to extrapolate some of their findings to human beings. As has been mentioned, if a human subject is truly resistant to hypertension, average amounts of salt in the diet will not affect his resistance. If on the other hand, he has a hereditary susceptibility to essential hypertension, he may be able to avoid hypertension entirely by lifetime adherence to a low-salt intake. However, if he eats 10 gm of salt daily, his hereditary predisposition will become apparent as his blood pressure gradually begins to rise into the hypertensive range.

Early prehistoric man is thought to have been a sodium-deficient herbivore, desperate for dietary sodium in order to survive and multiply. The taste receptors for salt in the human tongue are of interest in this context. Evolution has equipped us to cope with sodium deficiency rather than with sodium excess. It is no wonder, then, that certain of us become hypertensive when we eat excessive amounts of salt.

It is particularly easy to produce salt hypertension in young rats and is more difficult in adult rats. This brings up the fact that in the recent past, most commercial baby food had a very high salt content. Dahl et al. [11] were able to give hypertension to their susceptible rats by feeding them the baby food that is sold in grocery stores. Such salt-laden food is probably harmful to an infant who is susceptible to later hypertension. Another danger to infants is posed by the salt content of cow's milk, which has four times more sodium per milliliter than human milk.

Mechanism of Salt-Induced Hypertension

By what mechanism does salt feeding produce hypertension in susceptible rats or men? In susceptible rats, it is easy to produce hypertension by feeding a diet containing 8 percent sodium chloride [2], a situation reminiscent of that of the Japanese farmers. Such rats readily come into sodium balance, and it has been theorized that the hypertension results from damage to the kidney caused by the large amount of sodium excreted every day.

To test this proposition, we [12] fed the 8 percent sodium diet to two groups of rats. One group of 130 rats drank tap water ad lib. Another group of 111 rats had 0.01 percent of the thiazide diuretic Enduron in their drinking water. A control group of 35 rats ate a normal diet, with 0.3 percent sodium. These diet regimens were continued for 4¼ months.

As can be seen in Table 2-1, final blood pressures for the group on an 8 percent salt diet averaged 27 mm Hg higher than for the group with a normal intake, which is a 22 percent rise in pressure and statistically a higher significant difference. However, when a thiazide diuretic was combined with this same high sodium intake, the hypertension was completely prevented. If we consider all pressures above 140 as hypertensive, we see that both the group on a normal salt intake and the group on 8 percent sodium plus thiazide had a zero incidence of hypertension; without thiazide, the 8 percent salt diet produced a 48 percent incidence of hypertension.

Table 2-1. Effect of Thiazide on Sodium-Induced Hypertension

Diet	Final Blood Pressure (mm Hg)	Percent Above 140 (mm Hg)	Inulin Space (ml/100 gm)
8% NaCl (130 rats)	148 ↑	48 ↑	29.8 ↑
			(4.6% diff. in ECF)
	$p < .0001$	$p < .0001$	$p < .03$
8% NaCl plus thiazide (111 rats)	↓ 122	↓ 0	↓ 28.5
0.3% NaCl (35 rats)	121	0	28.0

In a separate group of rats we determined the inulin space as an index of extracellular fluid volume after eight days on these three regimens (Table 2-1). Rats on the 8 percent salt diet to which thiazide was added showed a 4.6 percent difference in extracellular fluid (ECF) volume, a significant drop ($p = .03$) from that of the rats fed an 8 percent salt diet without thiazide, and the addition of thiazide brought their ECF volume close to that of control rats on normal sodium intake. This study would indicate that the mere passage of sodium chloride through the renal tubular system does not necessarily cause hypertension. *A high sodium chloride intake may produce hypertension if it increases ECF volume. The same high intake produces no hypertension if ECF expansion is prevented.*

This brings us to question how a chronically high ECF volume, such as that produced by salt feeding, can bring on hypertension.

High Extracellular Fluid Volumes–High Blood Volume States
There are several situations in which the body has an inappropriately high ECF volume associated with a large "effective" blood volume. In this context I am not referring to the edema states of congestive heart failure, cirrhosis, or nephrosis, in which the total ECF volume is high and the "effective" blood volume is actually low, but rather to states with a high ECF volume and a high "effective" blood volume, in which we often find a high incidence of hypertension. These states are exemplified by mineralocorticoid excess and large salt intakes in the presence of renal disease.

If too much deoxycorticosterone is given to a rat, or if too much aldosterone emerges from a human renal adenoma, the kidney is induced to retain sodium and water until "escape" begins to occur. At this point, no further sodium will be retained, but the general level of body sodium and water is slightly elevated. Over a long period, this can produce hypertension in a susceptible animal.

Coleman and Guyton [13] studied the effects of giving large sodium loads to dogs with deficient renal function. They found that when dogs with only one-third of their normal renal mass were given 2 liters of saline a day to drink, there was an initial tendency toward sodium and water retention, and hypertension subsequently developed. We see this in patients with advanced renal parenchymal disease who are eating a large amount of salt. They commonly have high blood volumes and considerable hypertension. We also see this in uremic patients whose kidneys are almost totally destroyed by disease. They usually have hypertension when their ECF volume is elevated from dietary salt and water, but the hypertension usually disappears when the ECF volume is brought back to low normal levels by dialysis. This reversible change in arterial pressure may be repeated two times a week, coinciding with the dialysis cycle. Moreover, some patients with acute glomerulonephritis and marked sodium and water retention have a high blood and ECF volume and a high arterial pressure.

THE PROCESS OF AUTOREGULATION. In all these instances the veins could easily accommodate the modest elevation of blood volume. However, the extra volume will often increase venous filling pressure, which in turn will increase cardiac output. The higher cardiac output, of course, tends to increase arterial pressure. Moreover, a rise in cardiac output produced in this way induces tissue blood flows that are inappropriately high for metabolic needs. This situation would call forth an autoregulation of blood flow in many tissue beds; that is, an arteriolar vasoconstriction would occur to bring tissue flow back to normal levels. This would certainly be the case for the brain, muscle, gut, and kidney. In this autoregulatory response, most tissue beds would undergo arteriolar vasoconstriction, thereby raising the general peripheral resistance. The combination of the higher cardiac output and increased vasocontriction would tend to put the blood pressure even higher; and as the arterial pressure went higher, the cardiac output would gradually come back toward normal levels. After a time the cardiac output would be about normal, while the peripheral resistance and blood pressure would remain elevated. In this way, the underlying tendency to a higher cardiac output would be completely masked.

The higher arterial pressure, through the medium of pressure diuresis, would enhance the sodium and water output by the kidney in situations in which renal function was well preserved. This would tend to bring ECF volume somewhat closer to normal. However, if there were a renal abnormality, it would tend to preserve a slight ECF volume expansion. Most of the partially nephrectomized dogs of Coleman and Guyton [13] underwent just these changes. It is a very reasonable explanation of how a high ECF volume can bring about an arterial hypertension with peripheral vasoconstriction. Ultimately, the systemic peripheral arterioles will undergo a "waterlogging" [14] and thickening of their walls [15], just as we see in all hypertension. This arteriolar "waterlogging" and thickening will also occur in the renal afferent arteries and arterioles. Moreover, the process of thickening will then itself make a major contribution to the increased peripheral resistance, even though it was not the original cause of it [14, 15]. This general mechanism is probably operative in the hypertension of many azotemic and uremic patients.

Genetic Suseptibility and Extracellular Fluid Volume

Although the preceding formulation is reasonable as it stands, there must be additional elements necessary for the hypertension brought on by excessive ECF volume. Bartter gave 20 mg of deoxycorticosterone daily for three weeks to human volunteers and produced no hypertension. The ECF volume must have risen maximally at the end of one week, but no hypertension subsequently occurred. These subjects were resistant to hypertension in spite of the effect of mineralocorticoid on ECF volume. Similarly, Dahl et al. [11] injected deoxycorticosterone into his two strains of rats, one sensitive and one resistant to salt hypertension. The sensitive strain promptly became hypertensive, but the resistant strain did not. The deoxycorticosterone exerted its mineralocorticoid effect on the rats of the resistant strain and raised ECF volume a bit, but nevertheless hypertension did not ensue. In both instances, some genetic susceptibility is required before the high ECF volume will produce hypertension.

Muirhead [16] gave large saline loads to bilaterally nephrectomized rabbits and produced a sizable rise in blood pressure; but if fragments of renal medulla were implanted subcutaneously in these same nephrectomized rabbits, the same saline load would produce only a very small rise in blood pressure. Evidently, the fragments of renal medulla were releasing humoral agents (prostaglandins) that prevented the volume-induced hypertension. Moreover, some uremic patients have a normal arterial pressure, and ECF expansion does not produce a significant rise in blood pressure and peripheral resistance in some of this group. *Thus, increased ECF volume seems to bring about hypertension only in a susceptible subject.* Part of this susceptibility may be related to thickened arterioles. However, the explanation of susceptibility is still mainly an enigma.

Effect of Diuretics on Autoregulatory Mechanism

When thiazide drugs or spironolactone are given to patients, the arterial blood pressure is usually lowered, and the hypertensive process can be reversed. These diuretics produce a slight decrease in ECF volume, which decreases venous filling pressure and cardiac output. The autoregulatory response to this drop in output would bring about systemic arteriolar dilatation. The lower cardiac output and the vasodilatation should lower arterial blood pressure. This would amount to antihypertensive whole-body autoregulation, or reverse autoregulation. Such reverse autoregulation could also be a mechanism that partially accounts for the antihypertensive action of both propranolol and guanethidine. Both agents lower cardiac output, which could eventually induce a lowered peripheral resistance by reverse autoregulation. Thus, adaptation to a rise or a drop in ECF volume can ultimately influence the peripheral arteriole to enhance or reduce hypertension. One of the main antihypertensive actions of the kidneys is to excrete the daily sodium load without any tendency to a rise in ECF volume. Failure to do this encourages hypertension.

When blood pressure is successfully lowered in the treatment of clinical hypertension, plasma volume is also lowered. A low sodium intake is particularly effective in the treatment of the hypertension associated with renal parenchymal disease. This would be expected, since the diseased kidney usually exhibits an impairment of sodium excretion. With a normal salt intake in this situation, extracellular volume builds up before sodium balance is attained. Curtailing salt consumption would reduce the excretory load on the diseased kidney and thereby reduce

ECF volume somewhat. As has been mentioned, this should reduce hypertensive pressure levels.

Our experiments in rats have clearly demonstrated that if hypertensive kidneys are perfused at a normal pressure, they will excrete subnormal amounts of both sodium and water [12]. If this occurred in the human body, it would lead to sodium and water retention. Such sodium and water retention tends to produce and maintain the hypertensive state. Once a hypertensive level of inflow pressure is reached, the hypertensive kidneys then become capable of excreting a normal amount of sodium and water. This shift in the pressure-natriuresis curve would indicate that the hypertensive kidney needs a high arterial pressure for adequate sodium excretion. Any trend toward a normal blood pressure would be thwarted by sodium retention. Hypertension thus tends to be maintained.

Experiments at the University of Iowa have demonstrated the effects of salt feedings in human subjects. When young normotensive subjects are fed 400 mEq of salt for four weeks, their forearm flow goes up, their forearm vascular resistance goes down, and the blood pressure remains the same. When the same procedure is applied to young subjects with borderline hypertension, the forearm vascular resistance goes up instead of down, and arterial pressure rises. These very mild hypertensive subjects respond totally differently to a dietary salt load. Extracellular fluid volume increases in both groups, but only in those with borderline hypertension do both blood pressure and peripheral resistance rise. Heavy salt intake in susceptible persons may initiate the hypertension mechanism.

An important fact to remember is that the arteries of hypertensives have an increased sodium content per unit of dry weight [14]. This may add to the thickening of the artery wall, with a resulting increase in vascular resistance. It may also relate to increased vasoconstriction.

The Role of the Kidney in Hypertension

Richard Bright noted long ago that severe renal parenchymal disease was associated with the thickened left ventricle that accompanies hypertension. Moreover, the transplantation of a normal kidney into such patients with uremia and hypertension brings about a dramatic fall in the blood pressure to normal levels. Thus, we can be certain that the kidney plays a key role in some forms of hypertension. As mentioned previously, any renal disease that grossly retards the excretion of sodium is also apt to lead to hypertension. Narrowing of the renal artery to the remaining kidney after the other has been removed ultimately leads to sodium and water retention and a temporarily increased cardiac output [12, 14]. In part, this sodium and water retention undoubtedly helps to sustain the hypertension.

The Kidney's More Specific Prohypertensive Actions

There is definite evidence, however, that the kidney with a narrowed renal artery promotes hypertension in ways other than through volume expansion. In man and in the rat, hypertension will appear when only one renal artery is narrowed and the opposite kidney remains intact; in the rat, this occurs in the absence of any sodium and water retention [12]. In sheep, in fact, the narrowing of one renal artery with the opposite kidney intact actually promotes a loss of ECF volume, but the sheep nonetheless become hypertensive. When a Goldblatt clamp is removed from a lone renal artery, blood pressure promptly drops to normal, and the drop is not necessarily related to changes in fluid volume. Floyer [17] demonstrated in rats that volume changes were not necessary to achieve a reduction in blood pressure after freeing the compression of the renal artery. In the dog, an acute narrowing of a lone renal artery will ordinarily produce some hypertension within a few hours. Samuels and colleagues [18] showed that this early rise in blood pressure can be completely eliminated when an inhibitor to angiotensin I converting enzyme is infused at the time the renal artery is narrowed. This study indicates almost conclusively that the early rise in blood pressure after a narrowing of a renal artery is mediated by angiotensin and is not volume-dependent.

These experimental and clinical data have given us a reasonably clear picture of the mechanism of renovascular hypertension. As a result of the decreased pressure beyond the stenosed renal artery, the sequence of events occurs that is shown in Figure 2-1.

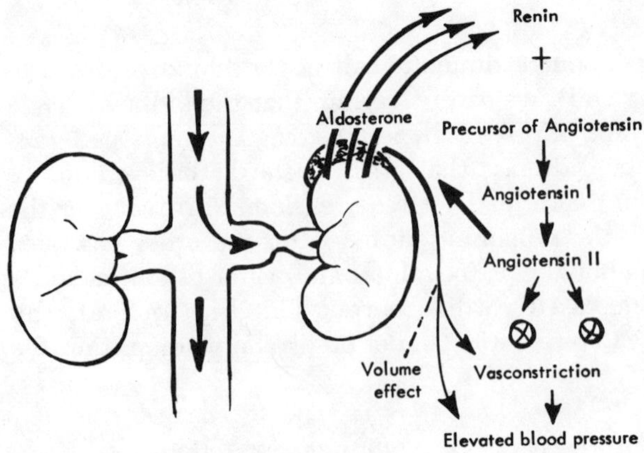

FIG. 2-1. Sequence of events in renovascular hypertension.

As a result of decreased flow to the juxtaglomerular apparatus, renin secretion is increased. Some sodium retention also occurs and there is reduced antihypertensive functioning of the kidney. Renin acts on a substrate to produce angiotensin I, which is converted in the lungs to angiotensin II, a potent vasoconstrictor agent. Vasoconstriction leads to an increase in peripheral resistance and a subsequent increase in blood pressure.

In addition, angiotensin II stimulates the adrenal cortex to increase aldosterone secretion. This in turn leads to an increase in sodium retention, plasma volume, and cardiac output, contributing to a further rise in blood pressure. Via a feedback mechanism, the higher blood pressure eventually acts to suppress the release of excess renin. Any drug that inhibits angiotensin therefore can break the cycle and prevent the rise in blood pressure. At present, the angiotensin antagonists are experimental drugs and are not available for clinical use.

While the role of angiotensin in chronic "renovascular hypertension" is not so clear-cut, there are data that do support its role in the pathogenesis of chronic two-kidney Goldblatt hypertension, or even in one-kidney hypertension if salt retention is prevented [19].

In the chronic phase, if sodium is available, volume expansion seems more important than renin in maintaining the hypertension in animals with one-kidney Goldblatt hypertension. However, if sodium is not available, the action of renin becomes the dominant mechanism. In either case, the blood pressure inexorably rises to hypertensive levels. Angiotensin also contributes to arteriolar narrowing in most cases of human malignant hypertension, since specific inhibtors of angiotensin II will bring the blood pressure back to normal [20].

The Kidney's Antihypertensive Actions

In addition to its prohypertensive features, such as the renin system, the kidney also possesses undoubted antihypertensive actions. Proof of this is found in the following: (1) removal of a contralateral kidney always intensifies unilateral Goldblatt hypertension in the dog; (2) removal of a kidney always worsens mineralocorticoid hypertension; (3) bilateral nephrectomy or severe renal parenchymal damage in man leads to hypertension. Transplantation of a good human kidney in such situations can completely relieve the hypertension.

Part of this antihypertensive effect may be just the facilitation of sodium diuresis. Loss of renal mass encourages some sodium and water retention, and this can lead to hypertension, as we have already indicated. Moreover, when many nephrons are absent, the sodium excretory burden is especially heavy on the few surviving ones. This extra burden somehow gradually promotes an additional rise in blood pressure. Moreover, there is considerable evidence that the kidney is capable of secreting antihypertensive humoral substances. The best evidence for this is Muirhead and colleagues' [16] implantation of renal medullary fragments under the skin of hypertensive rats and rabbits. These fragments survive and secrete materials that lower the blood pressure. We have confirmed this observation [21]. Moreover, when these implants are surgically removed, the blood pressure again climbs back to the previous hypertensive levels.

It has been determined that the interstitial cells from the implants contain substances belonging to the *prostaglandin* group of compounds. The E_2 prostaglandin, normally found in the renal inner medulla, is a potent antihypertensive substance and may account, at least in part, for the kidney's antihypertensive properties. A deficiency of interstitial-cell secretion in the kidney might lead to hypertension if this concept is correct. Zusman and colleagues [22] have found, for instance, that patients with essential hypertension have only 38 percent as much of A_2 prostaglandin (a possible product of E_2 prostaglandin) as normotensive subjects. These data correlate well with the findings of fewer lipid-containing granules in the interstitial cells of hypertensive animals. Of some clinical interest is the fact that these cells, when removed from animals and implanted under the skin of another animal, are capable of secreting large amounts of antihypertensive substances, including E_2 prostaglandin.

Urinary kallikrein, an additional humoral substance coming from the kidney, may also fit somewhere into the kidney's role in hypertension. Urinary kallikrein is produced locally in the kidney, appears abundantly in the urine, and can be easily measured there. Patients with essential hypertension have low levels of urinary kallikrein; even the children of hypertensive families appear to have low levels of urinary kallikrein [23]. Patients with Conn's adenomas have very high levels, and patients with Addison's disease have very low levels [23]. Kinins stimulate the secretion of E_2 prostaglandin by the kidney [24]. Urinary kallikrein seems to have a place in the total scheme, but its role is not yet well delineated.

From these pieces of information, we can conclude that the kidney has both a prohypertensive and an antihypertensive action. Nevertheless, whether kidney malfunction does or does not cause essential hypertension is still a moot point. We are particularly in doubt on this point because no specific renal disease is seen in early essential hypertension, and the levels of circulating renin are not elevated. To solve this problem, our best course is to consider the types of experimental hypertension that most closely resemble essential hypertension. These are conditions in which renal function is reasonably intact and in which there are no functional Goldblatt clamps to cause underperfusion of the renal parenchyma.

Role of the Kidney in Experimental Hypertension

One type of experimental hypertension that resembles essential hypertension can be termed *post-Goldblatt hypertension.* In this situation, a clip narrows one renal artery in a rat for a period of six to nine months, and the contralateral kidney remains untouched [25]. If the clip is removed from the artery, or if the clipped kidney is excised, the hypertension may nevertheless persist indefinitely. When Floyer [26] removed such a clip after several months, many of his rats remained hypertensive. He then divided these hypertensive rats into two groups. In one group he excised the previously clipped kidney, and the hypertension continued without any abatement. In the other group he excised the previously untouched kidney, and the elevated blood pressure levels promptly returned to normal. This was a clear indication that something occurring in the untouched kidney was causing the hypertension to persist. It could be inferred that vascular disease in the untouched kidney was acting like little Goldblatt clamps. However, if this were the case, a normal or increased number of juxtaglomerular granules should have been present in the kidney, just as in malignant hypertension. In actual fact, we found that the number of juxtaglomerular granules in the untouched kidney was only one-fourth of normal, indicating a reduced output of renin [25]. Hence, one is persuaded that in so-called post-Goldblatt hypertension, some condition in the untouched kidney, possibly unrelated to its cortical vascular disease, is the cause of the persistent hypertension.

Another type of experimental hypertension that resembles essential hypertension is that produced by a high salt intake. Dahl et al. [11] have shed much light on this type of hypertension by breeding one strain of rats highly susceptible to salt hypertension and another strain highly resistant to it. These two strains of rats have been compared in many ways, and it now begins to emerge that *the salt-sensitive rats are different primarily because the antihypertensive action of their kidneys is deranged.*

From available data, it seems clear that in the salt-sensitive rats some genetic defect in the kidneys promotes the acquisition of hypertension—a genetic defect that is absent in the salt-resistant rats, making them very resistant to most forms of hypertension.

Bianchi and Fox [27], in Milan, have produced a third form of experimental hypertension, working with spontaneously hypertensive rats they bred. When they transplant the "hypertensive" kidneys of these rats into normotensive control rats, the blood pressure of the normotensive recipients rises. When the kidneys of the normotensive control rats are transplanted into the spontaneously hypertensive rats, the blood pressure of the hypertensive recipients falls. Here again, there is strong evidence that the kidney in particular somehow determines the difference between hypertension and normal blood pressure, at least in these Milanese rats.

Speculations on the Role of Rat Kidney in Human Hypertension

Three types of experimental hypertension that closely resemble essential hypertension are all caused primarily by a disturbance in kidney function. Therefore, the best explanation for chronic established essential hypertension is that it, too, is caused primarily by a disordered kidney function, even though the aberration is not visible in tissue sections stained with hematoxylin and eosin. In essential hypertension, heredity dictates that there will be a greater and greater derangement of some specific antihypertensive component of renal function as life progresses. A lifelong high salt intake accelerates the deterioration of this specific antihypertensive function, and a low salt intake probably retards the rate of deterioration [3]. An inborn tendency toward an inappropriately high cardiac output would hasten the rate of deterioration, and hypertension itself may also accelerate it. Thus, we have the components of a vicious cycle, in which hypertension begets hypertension. When advanced renal parenchymal disease obviously destroys kidney tissue, it also accelerates the degradation of the renal antihypertensive function.

Even the hypertension of primary hyperaldosteronism probably works by this same mechanism. One can presume that when this situation continues for months and years, there is an accelerated degradation of the specific antihypertensive functions of the kidney, and eventually hypertension makes its appearance. When the offending aldosteronoma is removed, the kidney makes a partial comeback and extracellular fluid volume decreases, allowing the blood pressure to return to normal levels. If the deterioration of the specific renal function is severe enough, hypertension may continue indefinitely, even after the adenoma has been excised, as is seen in about a fourth of patients with aldosteronoma.

It will be of interest to see how close these speculations are to the facts that will emerge in the years to come.

Clinical Implications

Effect of Antihypertensive Drugs on Extracellular Volume

The mechanisms and principles derived from investigation of clinical and experimental hypertension help us in the management of hypertensive patients. If a generous intake of sodium chloride encourages the advent of hypertension, we have learned that a thiazide diuretic can overcome the effect of this extra intake of salt and can prevent the hypertension that results from it. This is undoubtedly one of the reasons that the thiazide diuretics by themselves can bring the blood pressure down to the normal range in half the patients with essential hypertension. The slight decrease in extracellular fluid volume that is brought about by thiazides is an important determinant of successful antihypertensive action. The same general principles also apply to the antihypertensive action of the diuretic aldosterone antagonist spironolactone.

We have also seen that the isolated kidney from rats with "post-salt" hypertension will definitely retain sodium and water when perfused with normal levels of inflow pressure. This same sort of thing happens in our patients who are given antihypertensive drugs such as hydralazine, diazoxide, methyldopa, guanethidine, and reserpine. When the blood pressure has been lowered by these drugs, and the kidney consequently retains sodium, the gradual accumulation of ECF volume tends to make the person resistant to the action of the antihypertensive drug, and the blood pressure begins to rise to the previous high level. This situation can be obviated if a diuretic drug is given in conjunction with the other antihypertensive agents. If this has been done, when the drug lowers the blood pressure, and the kidney begins to retain sodium, the diuretic overcomes the tendency for sodium retention, and the antihypertensive drug continues to be effective. The thiazide drugs and spironolactone are both effective in maintaining the potency of other antihypertensive agents.

The *azotemic patient* with hypertension tends to retain sodium, which very often produces a rise in arterial pressure. Part of this rise is possibly related to the tendency for cardiac filling pressure and cardiac output to increase, thus activating whole-body autoregulation. This sequence of events can be obviated to a certain extent by reducing the intake of sodium in such patients to no more than 50 or 60 mEq per day. If this is done, the intake of sodium better matches the impaired ability of the kidney to excrete sodium, and the tendency to an elevated extracellular fluid volume is reduced. This definitely reduces the tendency for an elevation of blood pressure in such patients and also makes them much more susceptible to antihypertensive drugs. Moreover, it decreases the likelihood of potassium abnormalities.

A tendency to a higher cardiac output may also be a factor in the rise in blood pressure in azotemic patients. This can be somewhat obviated by the use of beta-blocking drugs such as propranolol. The combination of a low sodium intake and propranolol can be effective in controlling the elevated blood pressure of moderately azotemic patients. The additional use of diuretic agents such as thiazides and spironolactone may also be helpful in slightly encouraging some diuresis in these patients. But, it may be necessary to use these drugs in conjunction with more powerful diuretics such as furosemide.

Whenever diuretic agents are used in the azotemic patient the electrolytes should be checked repeatedly and carefully to detect any early signs of a derangement of electrolyte pattern. If any early indications of such derangement occur, the pattern of diuretic administration may have to be altered. Furosemide provides a powerful diuretic action of brief duration. The sodium removal can then be subsequently maintained with the use of longer-acting diuretics, such as the thiazides or spironolactone.

Action of Antihypertensive Drugs on Renin

In certain types of severe or malignant hypertension in patients with or without renal insufficiency, there may be elevated levels of circulation renin, and the high angiotensin levels that result play a direct and important role in maintaining the elevation of blood pressure. (This has been conclusively demonstrated with the use of the angiotensin-blocking agents.)

In such patients a beta-blocking agent such as propranolol reduces the secretion of renin by the juxtaglomerular cells, thereby bringing renin levels down to normal. Such lowering of renin activity can have a very powerful effect in bringing the blood pressure closer to normal levels, provided that ECF volume is kept slightly below normal and not allowed to expand. In the hypertensive patient who has a normal level of circulating renin, propranolol can again be helpful in lowering blood pressure, partly through a reduction in renin level and partly through a decrease in cardiac output, with subsequent reduction in peripheral resistance through the mechanism of "reverse whole-body autoregulation."

The other very important action of beta-blocking drugs in such patients relates to their combination with diuretic agents, such as thiazides and spironolactone. When either of these diuretic agents are given to the typical patient with moderate hypertension, they will invariably cause a distinct rise in circulating renin level. If propranolol is given in conjunction with these diuretic agents, it lowers the level of circulating renin as the action of the diuretic agent continues. It thus allows the beneficial effect of diuretic action without the adverse effect of a rise in circulating renin level.

The Role of Diet

The thiazide diuretics are always more effective if they are combined with a low sodium intake. With such a combination, the dosage of the thiazide can be reduced, which tends to reduce some of the side effects of thiazides. A really large intake of salt can actually overcome the antihypertensive action of modest thiazide dosage. A reduction of salt intake is not so easy to bring about as one might think, since Langford has shown that patients on thiazide diuretic agents tend to have a much stronger appetite for salt in the diet. This is not an unexpected biologic result, since it has been known for many years that rats placed on a low-sodium diet have an intensified appetite for salt.

Effect of Sympathetic Blockers

Drugs such as guanethidine partly lower blood pressure by enlarging the capacity of the veins, thereby permitting pooling of blood in the upright posture, with consequent decreases in cardiac output. Over a long period of time, this may result in some dilatation of the peripheral arterioles by the mechanism of reverse whole body autoregulation.

Renovascular Hypertension

Hypertension due to a narrowed renal artery (Goldblatt hypertension) is the most difficult of all to treat with drugs. In a patient with Goldblatt hypertension there is a tendency both for ECF volume and the level of circulating renin to be elevated. Both these factors tend to raise the arterial pressure. Moreover, there is evidence that beyond the already demonstrated actions of volume and renin, there are other mechanisms that are important in the elevation of blood pressure. In the treatment of such patients it is far better, if feasible, to bring about a complete correction of the condition, either by surgical repair of the narrowing of the renal artery or, if this cannot be done, by removal of the stenotic kidney.

Hunt and Strong [28], in a carefully studied series, noted that patients with definite Goldblatt hypertension treated medically fared much worse in terms of life expectancy than those who received surgical treatment. It was very difficult to reduce the blood pressures of those on medical treatment to the upper limits of the normal range, but the pressures of many whose surgical treatment was successful were reduced well down into the normal range. This difference alone can be decisive in terms of subsequent life expectancy.

Moreover, treating Goldblatt hypertension is not the same as treating severe hypertension associated with renal arteriolar sclerosis and necrosis. When the blood pressure in malignant hypertension is lowered by drugs, the lesions in the arterioles of the kidney usually heal. Many of the thousands of tiny "Goldblatt" narrowings are opened up and the renin levels may come down into the normal range. On the other hand, when the same drugs are used to treat the narrowing of the main renal artery, there is no cure of the narrowing, and the kidney must fight every inch of the way to bring the blood pressure back up to elevated levels. In a patient with a mild narrowing of a renal artery, it is possible that antihypertensive drugs can bring about a satisfactory drop in pressure. However, if the narrowing is severe, the patient may be resistant to drug therapy and may require very large doses to bring the pressure down to the upper end of the normal range. The doses may have to be so high that side effects may be intolerable. This is another reason why surgical therapy is far preferable to medical therapy in tight stenosis of the renal artery.

In clinical practice one often sees hypertensive patients in whom a narrowing of a renal artery is demonstrated by arteriogram, but many of these patients actually have essential hypertension with a subsequent development of a plaque in a renal artery. Often in these cases the seeming stenosis of the artery is playing virtually no part in causing the hypertension. Such patients may be very susceptible to a lowering of blood pressure with the usual antihypertensive drugs. In a true case of hypertension due entirely to a stenosis of a renal artery, it is difficult to lower the blood pressure with the thiazide drugs used alone.

General Plan for the Diagnosis of Goldblatt Hypertension

Hypertension due to renal artery stenosis should be suspected in any of the following situations:

1. Onset of diastolic hypertension under age 30.
2. Presence of a systolic-diastolic abdominal bruit.
3. Sudden acceleration of long-standing normal blood pressure or mild hypertension to severe hypertension, or acceleration of essential hypertension.
4. Onset of hypertension following flank pain or injury.

The work-up for the diagnosis can include an intravenous urogram with minute-by-minute films during the early phases. If one kidney is more than 1.5 cm shorter than the other, this may be a sign of a stenosed renal artery. The findings suggestive of renovascular hypertension are as follows:

1. Difference in kidney size: difference of 1.5 cm or more in length, renal atrophy (difference in width), or both.
2. Delayed opacification of "ischemic" kidney.
3. Less than normally distended renal pelvis: "delicate" calyces.
4. Increased concentration of dye in late films of "ischemic" side.

A definitive examination would include an aortic arteriogram and even injecting the contrast material directly into a renal artery.

The other part of the diagnostic procedure is a renin evaluation, which can be done on another day. The main principle underlying this procedure is that an abrupt switch from suppression to sudden, strong stimulation of renin release will increase the chances of discovering a stenosed renal artery by eliciting great renin release from the stenosed kidney but not from the contralateral kidney with an open renal artery. The procedure involves taking the patient off all drugs except guanethidine and feeding him 200–300 mEq of sodium chloride each day for about three weeks. Then he is brought into the hospital and given chlorthalidone (Hygroton), 100 mg every 8 hours for three successive days, along with a diet containing only 10 mEq of sodium chloride per day. This combination produces a massive stimulation of renin release. On the morning of the third day of this program, renin levels are obtained in plasma from the left and right renal veins and from any artery or from the vena cava below the renal veins (in which the blood is similar to arterial blood). The concentration of renin in arterial plasma is subtracted from the concentration in the plasma in each renal vein to estimate roughly the amount of renin that each kidney contributes to the plasma that enters it. In a classic case of unilateral renal artery stenosis, the stenosed kidney adds much renin to the arterial blood entering it, while the opposite kidney adds none at all. Such a pattern augurs well for a successful surgical outcome.

Some investigators have shortened and simplified this procedure by administering 80 mg of furosemide to a patient on a moderate salt intake and checking renin levels 4–5 hours later, after a significant diuresis.

If peripheral renin levels are high, there is a far greater likelihood that the anatomical narrowing of the renal artery is actually producing the hypertension.

In *summary*, salt and extracellular fluid volume excess play a significant role in both the genesis and perpetration of human hypertension. These factors are more important in genetically susceptible persons than in those resistant to hypertension. The role of the kidney is twofold: (1) to aid in regulating salt and water excretion and extracellular fluid volume; (2) to stimulate renin production, which leads to angiotensin production and stimulation of increased aldosterone (the latter mechanism is operative in human renovascular hypertension, which is reversible in about 50–60 percent of patients following surgical correction of the narrowed renal artery); (3) to exert an antihypertensive action to keep blood pressure within a normal range.

References

1. Kempner, W. Treatment of kidney disease and hypertensive vascular disease with rice diet. *N.C. Med. J.* 5:125, 1944.
2. Meneely, G. R., et al. Chronic sodium chloride toxicity in the albino rat. II. Occurrence of hypertension and of a syndrome of edema and renal failure. *J. Exp. Med.* 98:71, 1953.
3. Prior, I. A. M., and Evans, J. G. Sodium intake and blood pressure in Pacific populations. *Isr. J. Med. Sci.* 5:608, 1969.
4. Page, L. B., Damon, A., and Moellering, R. C. Antecedents of cardiovascular disease in six Solomon Islands societies. *Circulation* 49:1132, 1974.
5. Shaper, A. G., et al. Environmental effects on the body build, blood pressure, and blood chemistry of nomadic warriors serving in the army in Kenya. *East Afr. Med. J.* 46:282, 1969.
6. Moser, M. Epidemiology of hypertension with particular reference to racial susceptibility. *Ann. N.Y. Acad. Sci.* 84:989, 1960.
7. Takahashi, E., et al. The geographical distribution of cerebral hemorrhage and hypertension in Japan. *Hum. Biol.* 29:139, 1957.
8. Dahl, L. K., and Love, R. A. Etiologic role of sodium chloride intake in essential hypertension in humans. *J. A. M. A.* 164:397, 1957.
9. Gifford, R. W., Jr. Personal communication.
10. Tobian, L., Ishii, M., and Duke, M. Relationship of cytoplasmic granules in renal papillary interstitial cells to "post-salt" hypertension. *J. Lab. Clin. Med.* 73:309, 1969.
11. Dahl, L. K., Heine, M., and Tassinari, L. Effects of chronic excess salt ingestion: Role of genetic factors in both DOCA-salt and renal hypertension. *J. Exp. Med.* 118:605, 1963.
12. Tobian, L., Coffee, K., and McCrea, P. Contrasting exchangeable sodium in rats with different types of Goldblatt hypertension. *Am. J. Physiol.* 217:458, 1969.
13. Coleman, T. G., and Guyton, A. C. Hypertension caused by salt loading in the dog. III. Onset transients of cardiac output and other variables. *Circ. Res.* 25:153, 1969.

14. Tobian, L., and Binion, J. T. Tissue cations and water in arterial hypertension. *Circulation* 5:754, 1952.
15. Folkow, D. The haemodynamic consequences of adaptive structural changes of the resistance vessels in hypertension. *Clin. Sci.* 41:1, 1971.
16. Muirhead, E. E., et al. The renal medulla as an antihypertensive organ. *J. Lab. Clin. Med.* 76:641, 1970.
17. Floyer, M. A. Further studies on the mechanism of experimental hypertension in the rat. *Clin. Sci.* 14:163, 1955.
18. Samuels, A. I., et al. The regulation of pressure by the renin-angiotensin system. *Fed. Proc.* 32:380, 1973.
19. Brunner, H. R., et al. Hypertension of renal origin. Evidence for two different mechanisms. *Science* 174:1344, 1971.
20. Brunner, H. R., et al. Hypertensive effects of angiotensin II blockade in man: Comparison with propranolol. *Circulation* 48:72, 1973.
21. Tobian, L., and Azar, S. Antihypertensive and other functions of the renal papilla. *Trans. Assoc. Am. Physicians* 84:281, 1971.
22. Zusman, R., et al. Prostaglandin A concentrations in plasma of normal and hypertensive humans. *J. Clin. Invest.* 59:93a, 1973.
23. Margolius, H., et al. Urinary kallikrein and aldosterone in essential hypertension. *Circulation* 48:83, 1973.
24. Lonigro, A. J., et al. Modification of the renal vasodilator action of bradykinin by an inhibitor of prostaglandin synthesis. *Fed. Proc.* 31:545, 1972.
25. Tobian, L., and Ishii, M. Interstitial cell granules and solutes in renal papilla in post-Goldblatt hypertension. *Am. J. Physiol.* 217:1699, 1969.
26. Floyer, M. A. The effect of nephrectomy and adrenalectomy upon the blood pressure in hypertensive and normotensive rats. *Clin. Sci.* 10:405, 1951.
27. Bianchi, G., and Fox, U. Die Bedeutung der Niere beim Hochdrunk spontanhypertensiver Ratten. *Ther. Woche* 23:4205, 1973.
28. Hunt, J. C., and Strong, C. G. Renovascular Hypertension—Mechanisms, Natural History and Treatment. In Laragh, J. H. (Ed.), *Hypertension Manual.* Dun-Donnelley, New York, 1974. P. 509.

3. Low Renin Hypertension*

J. Caulie Gunnells, Jr., and William L. McGuffin, Jr.

Low or suppressed plasma renin activity (PRA) was first described in association with primary hyperaldosteronism in 1964 by Conn et al. [1], who suggested that low plasma renin activity is one of the essential diagnostic criteria for primary hyperaldosteronism. They also pointed out that renin measurements were useful in the screening evaluation of hypertensive patients in the search for the diagnosis of primary hyperaldosteronism. When PRA was measured under carefully controlled conditions, low or suppressed PRA was observed in approximately 20–25 percent of their selected hypertensive population. This finding, together with the high incidence of adrenal abnormalities that had been reported in postmortem studies of patients with hypertension, led to the suggestion that a normokalemic form or variant of "classic" primary hyperaldosteronism might exist and could include as many as 20 percent of hypertensive patients otherwise classified as having benign essential hypertension [2].

In the following year, Conn and co-workers [3] described a patient with hypertension, suppressed PRA, normal serum potassium levels, and an elevated aldosterone excretion in whom an adrenal adenoma had been found at surgery and who became normotensive when the adenoma was removed.

For several years following these initial reports, many other investigators measured PRA in large numbers of hypertensive

* This work was supported in part by Training Grant HL05848, Renal Division, and CRU Grant MOIRR30 from the National Institutes of Health.

patients, selected and unselected, finding low or suppressed levels of PRA in 10–43 percent. However, in only a relatively small number of these patients was the diagnosis of primary aldosteronism actually established [4–12], which led several investigators to suggest that low plasma renin activity was a nonspecific finding unrelated to abnormalities of adrenal structure or function [4, 13].

Between 1969 and 1971, several investigators made preliminary observations suggesting that low renin hypertension was different from the usual variety of benign essential hypertension and was related pathogenetically to the adrenal gland [10, 11, 14]. In 1969, Woods et al. [14] documented that aminogluthethimide, an inhibitor of adrenal steroidogenesis, produced a reduction of blood pressure in 6 of 9 patients with suppressed renin activity and normal or low aldosterone levels. In our own laboratories [10], we observed a reduction in blood pressure following subtotal adrenalectomy in 4 of 6 patients with low PRA and normal aldosterone excretion rates. Pathologic abnormalities in the adrenal gland were found in 5 of these patients of which one was a single adenoma. Moreover, postoperative PRA studies in these patients demonstrated a return of renin responsiveness. The final set of observations came from Spark and Melby in 1971 [11], who found that 8 patients with low PRA and low aldosterone secretion rates responded to high-dose (400 mg per day) spironolactone therapy with a normalization of blood pressure and significant weight loss. This was in contrast to 15 patients with normal PRA who failed to show an appreciable weight or blood pressure reduction in response to similar doses of spironolactone over a five-week period.

It has become clear in the several years since these observations were reported that hypertension associated with low PRA is a feature of a spectrum of disorders including: (1) primary aldosteronism with either adenoma or hyperplasia; (2) various other forms of mineralocorticoid excess; (3) low renin essential hypertension with no easily definable abnormality in mineralocorticoid production, but in which the hypertension seems volume-dependent; and (4) several other miscellaneous conditions.

The observations that have been cited have led to controversy about the clinical and laboratory criteria for establishing the low renin state, its pathophysiologic mechanisms, the indications and modalities for treatment of the associated hypertension, and its prognosis. Here, we will review and, it is hoped, clarify some recent developments that have been the source of controversy in the syndrome of low renin hypertension.

Low renin hypertension is characterized by the presence of hypertension in association with a failure to demonstrate an appropriate rise in PRA in response to stimuli (posture, sodium restriction, and pharmacologic agents) that consistently stimulate a rise in PRA in other hypertensive patients or normal subjects [6, 9–11, 15, 16].*

In an investigation of renin responsiveness in 134 hypertensive patients from our own laboratory (Fig. 3-1 and Table 3-1) we found a 26 percent incidence of suppressed PRA. In this study a five-day period of sodium restriction (10 mEq per day), plus diuretics on the fourth day, was used to stimulate PRA. These results are comparable to those reported by others using a variety of maneuvers known to provoke an increase in PRA. The limitations of this somewhat lengthy approach to the stimulation of renin release have been circumvented in part by the out patient administration of "loop" diuretics such as furosemide (40–80 mg, orally or intravenously, depending on the specific protocol employed, with measurement of PRA before and 4–5 hours following the administration of furosemide, as well as some assessment of urinary Na^+ excretion prior to diuretic administration). The failure of patients to respond to such maneuvers with an appropriate increase in PRA has been judged to be evidence for the low renin state. When the results of this approach have been compared with those in previous studies in which dietary sodium restriction was used, there has been generally good agreement. Thus, it is now accepted by

* The kidney normally increases its secretion of renin in response to a decrease in pressure-flow that is sensed in the juxtoglomerular area (afferent arteriole to the glomerulus). Any reduction of pressure from a systemic loss of blood, congestive heart failure, salt depletion, or the upright position will normally cause a rise in renin unless it is suppressed by excessive amounts of mineralocorticoid. Most investigators have recognized the difficulty of distinguishing low levels of renin activity in hypertensive patients on an ad lib. sodium intake.

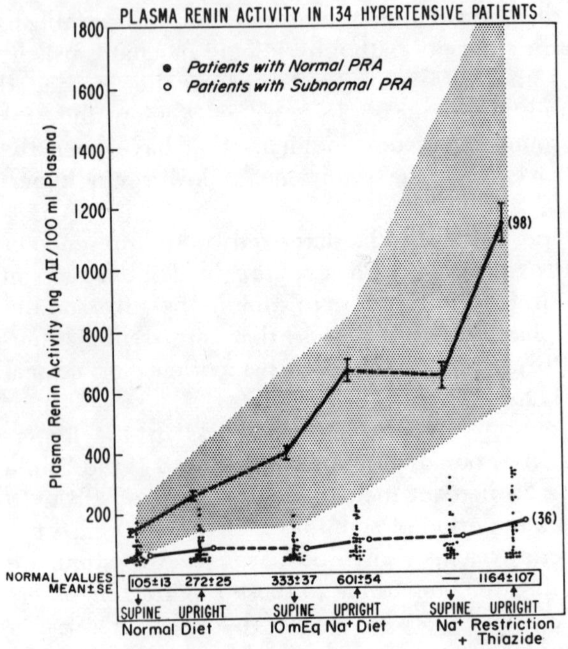

FIG. 3-1. Plasma renin activity (PRA) measurements in 134 hypertensive patients on a normal diet and following dietary sodium restriction alone and the subsequent administration of diuretics. The shaded area corresponds to the range of PRA values obtained in normal subjects on a similar protocol. The upper line overlying the shaded area reflects the average PRA of the 98 hypertensive subjects who responded to these maneuvers with an appropriate increase in PRA, as compared with normal subjects. The individual dots and the lower line (mean value) represent the PRA results in the 36 patients (26 percent) who were judged to have suppressed or subnormal PRA, defined in this study as failure to increase PRA in the upright position on the fourth day of Na+ restriction alone (urinary Na+ excretion < 40 mEq per 24 hours) or on the fifth day after the administration of diuretic to at least the lowest level of PRA observed in normal subjects under similar conditions of study.

most investigators that the use of furosemide to demonstrate the low renin state is a valid diagnostic maneuver. Although this simpler technique has led to a more frequent definition of the low renin hypertensive state, careful attention must be paid to such details as Na+ balance, prior or simultaneous drug therapy, and so on, for proper interpretation.

Brunner et al. [17, 18] and Mroczek et al. [19] have related

Table 3-1. Mean Plasma Renin Activity (PRA) in ng AII per 100 ml of Plasma in Normotensive and Hypertensive Subjects Studied Under Standardized Protocol Conditions to Detect Low or Suppressed PRA[a]

Subjects	Normal Diet[b]		10 mEq Na+ Diet[c]		10 mEq Na+ Diet plus Diuretic[d]
	Supine	Upright	Supine	Upright	Upright
Normotensive	105	272	333	601	1,164
Hypertensive					
Normal PRA	141	261	398	667	1,145
Low or subnormal PRA	60	82	63	114	133

[a] Number of subjects: normotensive, 16; hypertensive, 134 (98 with normal PRA, 36 with low PRA).
[b] Normal diet: 180 mEq Na+ and at least 100 mEq K+.
[c] Plasma obtained on day 4 of 10 mEq Na+ diet.
[d] Oral hydrochlorothiazide, 50 mg × 2 on day 4; plasma obtained on day 5.

PRA and aldosterone secretion rates to 24-hour urinary sodium excretion, thereby dividing hypertensive patients into low, normal, and high renin subgroups. The division into renin subgroups based on the renin methodology and the criteria of these investigators is not definitive unless urinary sodium excretion determined at the time of renin measurement is *less than* 150 mEq per 24 hours.

Physiologic Variables Affecting Renin Levels

It is important to be aware of some of the currently known variables that may affect levels of renin activity in general. Among these variables are age, sex, and race: plasma renin activity and aldosterone decrease with advancing age [20, 21]; in general, PRA is lower in females than in males [19]; and in most studies, PRA is observed to be lower in blacks [5, 8, 19] than in whites and other racial groups. Therefore, in evaluating a hypertensive patient with PRA measurements, one must compare the values obtained with the PRA in age-, sex-, and race-matched controls. Failure to do so may not be a major source of error, but it is one of which the physician must be aware.

It is also important for the clinician to be cognizant of the large number of other variables that may alter renin release if he is to evaluate the results of PRA measurements accurately. (For a full review of renin physiology and its feedback control, the reader is referred to recent publications [16, 22, 38].) Some commonly recognized conditions associated with increased or decreased renin release are outlined in Table 3-2. If one is to avoid pitfalls in classifying hypertensive patients based on PRA measurements, careful attention must be paid to the status of sodium and potassium balance, posture, and current and past drug history, to mention only a few of the important variables. Many of the drugs used in hypertensive therapy inhibit renin secretion. These include propranolol [23] and other adrenergic blockers, methyldopa [24], reserpine, ganglionic blockers [25], and clonidine. Other drugs may stimulate renin secretion; these include spironolactone [26], other diuretics [10, 27], and several vasodilators such as diazoxide, nitroprusside, and hydralazine [28]. These drugs should be withdrawn for at least a two-week period before evaluating renin responsiveness.

Table 3-2. Conditions Associated with Increased or Decreased Renin Activity

Increased Renin Release	Decreased Renin Release
Upright posture	Supine posture
Na+ restriction (volume depletion)	Na loading (volume expansion)
K+ depletion	K+ administration
Stimulation of autonomic nervous system	Blockade of autonomic nervous system
Drugs	Drugs
Diuretics, including spironolactone	Propranolol
Diazoxide	Methyldopa
Nitroprusside	Reserpine
Hydralazine	Ganglionic blockers
	Clonidine

Of equal importance is some knowledge of the techniques employed by the laboratory performing the renin measurements. It should be demonstrated that the method employed is of sufficient sensitivity to detect the low levels of PRA known to exist in patients with low renin hypertension [29, 30].

Differential Diagnosis of Low Renin Hypertension

The differential diagnosis of low renin hypertension can be divided into the four broad subtypes or categories outlined in Table 3-3, namely, (1) elevated levels of aldosterone, (2) elevation of other mineralocorticoids, (3) low renin essential hypertension, and (4) a miscellaneous group with a variety of unrelated abnormalities.

Aldosterone Excess

Elevated levels of aldosterone either in plasma or urine have been found in 3–50 percent of patients with hypertension and low PRA. In most series, approximately 5–10 percent of patients with low renin activity have elevated levels of aldosterone, *giving an incidence of hyperaldosteronism in the overall hypertensive population of less than 3 percent.*

Table 3-3. Differential Diagnosis of Low Renin Hypertension

Aldosterone excess
Aldosterone-producing adenoma (APA)
Idiopathic hyperaldosteronism (IHA)
Indeterminate hyperaldosteronism (Ind A)
Glucocorticoid-suppressible hyperaldosteronism
Other mineralocorticoid excess
Congenital adrenal hyperplasia
11-β-Hydroxylase deficiency
17-α-Hydroxylase deficiency
Ectopic ACTH syndrome
Adrenal carcinoma
Isolated DOC excess
18-OH-DOC excess
Low renin essential hypertension
Miscellaneous conditions
Licorice ingestion
Liddle's syndrome
Parenchymal renal disease (occasionally)

Patients with low renin hypertension in association with elevated levels of aldosterone can be classified into four subgroups, as follows:

1. Aldosterone-producing adenomas (APA)
2. Idiopathic hyperaldosteronism (adrenal hyperplasia, [IHA])
3. Indeterminate hyperaldosteronism (adrenal hyperplasia)
4. Glucocorticoid-suppressible hyperaldosteronism (adrenal hyperplasia)

Differential diagnosis between these four categories is critically important because surgical removal of an adrenal adenoma is curative in most patients who have aldosterone-producing adenomas [31, 32]. However, adrenal surgery in bilateral adrenal hyperplasia, found in the remaining three types of hyperaldosteronism, does not, in most instances, correct the hypertension, unless a subtotal or total adrenalectomy is performed. The patient may therefore be left with his hypertension, requiring antihypertensive therapy, and often will need adrenal hormone replacement as well.

In general, *patients with aldosterone-producing adenomas have lower serum potassium levels, a greater elevation in aldosterone secretion, and lower PRA levels than patients in the other three groups.* However, in individual patients, these findings do not allow for clinical separation between the other forms of aldosterone excess. An initial step in the differential diagnosis of these conditions in patients with a suspected adenoma is to determine whether or not the excessive aldosterone production is suppressed by certain physiologic maneuvers. This may be accomplished by inducing volume expansion in the patient, either with saline loading [33, 34] or deoxycorticosterone acetate (DOCA) or fludrocortisone administration [3]. Fortunately, the number of patients that must be evaluated in this way is small.

INDETERMINATE HYPERALDOSTERONISM. In patients in the indeterminate category, aldosterone excess will be suppressed to normal by one of the volume-expanding maneuvers mentioned above. They will also exhibit some elevation in their

PRA and plasma aldosterone levels with upright posture. Plasma renin activity is easily elevated following one month of low-dose spironolactone therapy (100 mg per day) and is associated with a fall in blood pressure.

ADENOMAS AND IDIOPATHIC HYPERALDOSTERONISM. In patients with idiopathic hyperaldosteronism (adrenal hyperplasia) and in those with aldosterone-producing adenoma, the volume-expanding maneuvers will not suppress aldosterone levels. However, those with idiopathic hyperaldosteronism may exhibit an increase in PRA and plasma aldosterone levels with upright posture. Patients with adenomas, on the other hand, fail to demonstrate an increase in PRA and aldosterone levels by this maneuver, and, paradoxically, plasma aldosterone may decrease. Another differential point between these two forms of hyperaldosteronism is that with spironolactone in moderate doses (200 mg per day) for one month, PRA will usually increase in patients with hyperplasia, but not in patients with classic Conn's syndrome (adenoma). However, with 400 mg per day, the blood pressure of both will be decreased [35, 36]. Ultimately, adrenal hyperplasia and adenoma are differentiated by actually identifying the adenoma by means of either adrenal venography [37] or iodocholesterol scanning [38] of the adrenal gland in conjunction with the identification of differential levels of plasma aldosterone from adrenal vein effluent [39].

GLUCOCORTICOID-SUPPRESSIBLE HYPERALDOSTERONISM. This form of hyperaldosteronism is extremely rare, with only 6 cases having been reported to date. Of the 6 patients, 5 were children, with two from the same family. These patients also usually have elevated levels of 18-hydroxycorticosterone or corticosterone. No enzymatic defect has been established in these patients to date. The hypertension and hypokalemia is easily corrected by low doses of dexamethasone therapy.

Obviously, the process of differentiating the various types of hyperaldosteronism is a complex, time-consuming, and expensive one; and, as previously noted, it is rarely necessary in the routine management of the vast number of hypertensive patients. Since the majority can be well controlled with carefully selected medical therapy, the number of patients identified as in need of extensive diagnostic testing should be small with appropriate application of screening maneuvers (e.g., hypokalemia, initially low PRA, benign hypertension).

Mineralocorticoid Excess

Other forms of mineralocorticoid hypertension (Table 3-3) are being discovered or described with increasing frequency as methods for measuring the levels of these hormones become more widely used. Non-aldosterone mineralocorticoids, which are capable of producing sodium retention and volume expansion and have been associated with hypertension, are deoxycorticosterone (DOC), corticosterone (compound B), and 18-hydroxydeoxycorticosterone (18-OH-DOC).

Several types of congenital adrenal hyperplasia (enzymatic defects in adrenal steroidogenesis) are clinically recognizable as virilizing syndromes or as primary amenorrhea in the female or pseudohermaphroditism in the male. In these cases, suppression of adrenocorticotropin (ACTH) with glucocorticoids will correct the hypertension as well as the electrolyte abnormalities.

Elevated levels of DOC alone have been reported in 6 of 21 patients with low renin hypertension [40]. These patients showed no evidence of neoplasia. Their hypertension was corrected with spironolactone. However, dexamethasone treatment was ineffective, suggesting that the elevated levels of DOC were not ACTH-dependent.

Recently, attention has been directed to a relatively low-potency human mineralocorticoid, 18-OH-DOC, reported to be elevated in 10 of 30 low renin hypertensive patients by Melby et al. [41]. In one patient treated with dexamethasone, blood pressure returned to normal, suggesting that this mineralocorticoid was under ACTH control. The adrenal abnormality in most of these patients was hyperplasia, although two had adrenal adenomas. In those with hyperplasia, dexamethasone reduced the blood pressure, and adrenalectomy was similarly effective in normalizing the pressure. Melby et al. have suggested that approximately 15 percent of a randomly selected group of low renin hypertensive patients will have marked elevation of 18-OH-DOC. In addition, they have described elevated levels of this mineralocorticoid in patients with otherwise classic forms of primary hyperaldosteronism. It is of interest that Genest and co-workers [42] found elevated levels of 18-OH-DOC in over 60 percent of their patients with essential hypertension. The significance of these findings remains uncertain at the present time.

Low Renin Essential Hypertension

The largest category of patients with low renin hypertension have no identifiable abnormality in mineralocorticoid secretion. While the precise pathophysiologic mechanisms in this group of hypertensive patients has not been clearly established, certain observations have been made that suggest either mild abnormalities in mineralocorticoid control or renal handling of sodium such that a state of effective volume expansion exists in these patients [43, 44].

It was initially suggested that spironolactone, an inhibitor of mineralocorticoid activity, was a specific form of therapy for low renin hypertension [45], that other diuretics were less effective, and that spironolactone alone was relatively ineffective in patients with normal renin hypertension. More recent evidence has suggested that thiazide diuretics effectively lower blood pressure in patients with low renin essential hypertension [46], although some observers believe that the response to thiazide diuretics is quantitatively less than that seen with spironolactone at comparable dose levels.

While it has been clearly established that patients with primary hyperaldosteronism have increased plasma and extracellular fluid volumes, as well as increased exchangeable sodium space, in comparison with both normal subjects and patients with essential hypertension [47], conclusive evidence of similar abnormalities in low renin hypertension has not been presented. Reports from different investigators vary. Some claim a definite increase in blood volume or exchangeable sodium space, or both, in low renin as compared with normal renin hypertensive states. Others find no significant difference.

Although volume expansion comparable to that found in primary aldosteronism is clearly not present in low renin hypertension, the evidence does suggest a mild abnormality of volume expansion in many of these patients. Perhaps the most convincing argument for the proposition that volume excess is a primary pathophysiologic derangement in low renin hypertensive patients is their uniform response to diuretic administration, namely, significant weight loss and reduction in blood pressure as compared with normal renin hypertensive patients, who frequently respond but not so dramatically and often require additional sequential antihypertensive therapy.

Miscellaneous Conditions

A small group of patients with low renin hypertension have a variety of miscellaneous abnormalities. Included are patients who have ingested excessive amounts of licorice [48], resulting in hypokalemia and hypertension that may mimic primary aldosteronism, but in whom the abnormal compound has been identified as glycyrrhizic acid.

Some patients with parenchymal renal disease and renal insufficiency in association with hypertension have low PRA levels. A volume-dependent form of hypertension has been postulated based on normalization of blood pressure with ultrafiltration on hemodialysis. In contrast, patients who fail to respond to ultrafiltration have demonstrated high renin activity and have required renin-blocking agents or nephrectomy for control of hypertension.

Treatment of Low Renin (Essential) Hypertension

The mainstay of treatment in patients with low renin essential hypertension clearly involves the use of diuretic agents, which, in most of these patients, reduces the blood pressure to normal. As has been mentioned, relatively greater success has been reported with spironolactone than with thiazide diuretics alone, although more recent studies have demonstrated that many patients with low renin essential hypertension respond very well to the thiazide diuretics, and the response to spironolactone can no longer be utilized as a unique feature of the low renin hypertensive state. However, spironolactone has been particularly useful in the medical management of low renin hypertension with aldosterone excess (Conn's syndrome).

The use of spironolactone in all forms of low renin hypertension, by avoiding the well-known kaliuretic effect of thiazides, which may be enhanced in states of mineralocorticoid excess, minimizes the need for supplemental potassium. The negative features of spironolactone are the side effects that sometimes occur with its administration. These include gastrointestinal disturbances, such as persistent nausea, and menorrhagia and gynecomastia. In low renin essential hypertension these potential adverse effects are largely theoretical, since the doses that have been effective are generally low (100–200 mg per day), with a low incidence of side effects in comparison with those occurring with the high-dose spironolactone therapy (400 mg per day) previously recommended.

If diuretic agents alone are not successful in reducing blood pressure to normal, then standard antihypertensive drugs should be used, since they are effective in this group of patients. *Thus, low renin hypertension is treated in much the same manner as most other kinds of hypertension, and it is usually not necessary to establish a renin profile prior to treatment.*

The currently recognizable clinical entities associated with low renin activity, together with their mineralocorticoid defects and a proposed scheme for treatment, are outlined in Table 3-4.

Table 3-4. A Treatment Scheme for Low Renin Hypertension

	Low Renin Activity		Treatment		
				Medical	
Diagnosis	Aldo ↑	Aldo Nl or ↓	Surgical	Corticosteroid	Diuretic[a]
Conn's syndrome	X		X		X
Idiopathic hyperaldosteronism	X				X
17-α-Hydroxylase defect		X		X	
11-β-Hydroxylase defect		X		X	
18-OH-DOC		X		X	X
DOC excess		X			X
Low renin essential hypertension		X			X

[a] Spironolactone versus thiazide diuretics.

Prognosis in Low Renin Hypertension

Perhaps the greatest area of controversy in the syndrome of low renin hypertension has been generated by the report of Brunner, Sealey, and Laragh [17] that patients with low renin hypertension had fewer cerebrovascular accidents and myocardial infarctions than patients with normal or high renin hypertension. These investigators originally reported on 59 patients with low renin hypertension in whom no strokes or myocardial infarctions occurred, as contrasted with an 11 and 14 percent incidence in the normal and high PRA subgroups, respectively. Recently, Christlieb et al. [49] have reported data supporting this concept. The conclusions of Laragh's group relative to the benign nature of low renin hypertension is at variance with the more recently reported data from five other laboratories [19, 50–53]. The results of these five studies indicate that patients with low renin hypertension have an equal number of morbid cardiovascular events—myocardial infarction, cerebrovascular accidents, and congestive heart failure—as do patients with normal or high renin hypertension.

Laragh has observed that these investigators are studying a different group of hypertensive patients because they have not followed similar protocols of renin profiling. This argument may not be altogether applicable, particularly in view of the fact that Catt's group [19] followed procedures similar to those in the Laragh group's study, with the exception of minor variations in the technique of renin activity measurements. They found a similar incidence of low, normal, and high renin hypertensions in their primarily black population and documented an equal incidence of myocardial infarctions and cerebrovascular accidents in the three renin subgroups [19]. Furthermore, Genest and co-workers [53] have demonstrated that the risk of myocardial infarction or a cerebrovascular accident is more closely related to the level of diastolic blood pressure, level of renal function, and efficacy of control of the hypertension than it is to the level of renin activity. Similar conclusions were reached by Gulati et al. [51], who demonstrated an actual increase in the number of morbid events in their group of patients with low renin hypertension. However, in their study, the levels of blood pressure in patients with low renin hypertension were significantly higher than in those with normal or high renin hypertension.

The results of the Veterans Administration cooperative study [54, 55] on antihypertensive agents, in which a large number of unselected men with hypertension were followed for five years or more without reference to renin activity levels, have demonstrated the beneficial effect of blood pressure reduction in decreasing the number of morbid events in effectively treated hypertension.

The evidence seems conclusive that low renin hypertension is not necessarily a benign form of hypertension; that is, it is not different in terms of predisposing the patient to myocardial infarction, cerebrovascular accidents, and congestive heart failure than are other forms of hypertension, and that it should not be therapeutically ignored. It is clear that this hypertensive syndrome must be treated as vigorously as other forms of hypertension if the risk of morbid cardiovascular events is to be reduced.

Summary

Low renin hypertension comprises a spectrum of disorders ranging from primary aldosteronism to obvious disorders of other mineralocorticoids, as well as a variety of miscellaneous conditions. The largest group of patients with low renin hypertension have no clear abnormality in mineralocorticoid production. However, many lines of evidence suggest the critical role of volume excess in the pathogenesis of hypertension in these patients. More detailed physiologic studies must be carried out if the spectrum of pathophysiologic factors in low renin hypertension is to be completely understood, and such studies are in progress. However, evidence already available from the literature clearly indicates that low renin hypertension must be treated and that in most of these patients diuretic administration, either spironolactone or a thiazide diuretic, is usually effective in reducing blood pressure to normal levels. At present, there is little indication for routine renin profiles to be done prior to instituting antihypertensive therapy in typical hypertensive patients without complications.

References

1. Conn, J. W., Cohen, E. L., and Rovner, D. R. Suppression of plasma renin activity in primary aldosteronism: Distinguishing primary from secondary aldosteronism in hypertensive disease. *J. A. M. A.* 190:213, 1964.
2. Conn, J. W. Plasma renin activity in primary aldosteronism: Importance in differential diagnosis and in research of "essential" hypertension. *J. A. M. A.* 190:222, 1964.
3. Conn, J. W., et al. Normokalemic primary aldosteronism: A detectable cause of curable "essential" hypertension. *J. A. M. A.* 193:100, 1965.
4. Creditor, M. C., and Loschky, U. K. Incidence of suppressed renin activity and of normokalemic primary aldosteronism in hypertensive Negro patients. *Circulation* 38:1027, 1968.
5. Helmer, O. M., and Judson, W. E. Metabolic studies on hypertensive patients with suppressed plasma renin activity not due to hyperaldosteronism. *Circulation* 38:965, 1968.
6. Gunnells, J. C., et al. Plasma renin activity in healthy subjects and patients with hypertension. *Arch. Intern. Med.* 119: 232, 1967.
7. Fishman, L. M., et al. Incidence of primary aldosteronism in uncomplicated essential hypertension. *J. A. M. A.* 205:497, 1968.
8. Channick, B. J., Adlin, E. V., and Marks, A. D. Suppressed plasma renin activity in hypertension. *Arch. Intern. Med.* 123: 131, 1969.
9. Jose, A., and Kaplan, N. M. Plasma renin activity in the diagnosis of primary aldosteronism. *Arch. Intern. Med.* 123:141, 1969.
10. Gunnells, J. C., et al. Hypertension, adrenal abnormalities, and alterations in plasma renin activity. *Ann. Intern. Med.* 73:901, 1970.
11. Spark, R. F., and Melby, J. C. Hypertension and low plasma renin activity: presumptive evidence for mineralocorticoid excess. *Ann. Intern. Med.* 75:831, 1971.
12. Streeten, D. H. P., et al. Studies of the renin angiotension-aldosterone system in patients with hypertension and in normal subjects. *Am. J. Med.* 46:844, 1969.
13. Kaplan, N. M. Commentary on incidence of primary aldosteronism: Current estimations based on objective data. *Arch. Intern. Med.* 123:152, 1969.
14. Woods, J. W., et al. Effect of an adrenal inhibitor in hypertensive patients with suppressed renin. *Arch. Intern. Med.* 123:366, 1969.
15. Cohen, E. L., Rovner, D. R., and Conn, J. R. Postural augmentation of plasma renin activity. *J. A. M. A.* 197:973, 1966.

16. Stein, J. H., and Ferris, T. F. The physiology of renin. *Arch. Intern. Med.* 131:860, 1973.
17. Brunner, H. R., Sealey, J. E., and Laragh, J. H. Renin as a risk factor in essential hypertension: More evidence. *Am. J. Med.* 55:295, 1973.
18. Laragh, J. H., et al. Renin, angiotension and aldosterone system in pathogenesis and management of hypertensive vascular disease. *Am. J. Med.* 52:633, 1972.
19. Mroczek, W. J., Finnerty, F. A., and Catt, K. J. Lack of association between plasma-renin and history of heart attack or stroke in patients with essential hypertension. *Lancet* 2:464, 1973.
20. Tuck, M., et al. Relation of age, diastolic pressure and known duration of hypertension to presence of low renin essential hypertension. *Am. J. Cardiol.* 32:637, 1973.
21. Sambhi, M. P., Crane, M. G., and Genest, J. Essential hypertension: New concepts about mechanisms. *Ann. Intern. Med.* 79:411, 1973.
22. Davis, J. O. The control of renin release. *Am. J. Med.* 55:333, 1973.
23. Bühler, F. R., et al. Propranolol inhibition of renin secretion. A specific approach to diagnosis and treatment of renin-dependent hypertensive disease. *N. Engl. J. Med.* 287:1209, 1972.
24. Mohammed, S., et al. Effect of methyldopa on plasma renin activity in man. *Circulation* 35:593, 1969.
25. Kameko, Y., et al. Effect of ganglion-blocking agents on renin release in hypertensive patients. *Circ. Res.* 27:97, 1970.
26. Spark, R. F., and O'Hare, C. M. Low renin hypertension. Restoration of normotension and renin responsiveness. *Arch. Intern. Med.* 133:205, 1974.
27. Bourgoignie, J. J., Catanzaro, F. J., and Perry, H. M., Jr. Renin-angiotension-aldosterone systems during chronic thiazide therapy of benign essential hypertension. *Circulation* 37:27, 1968.
28. Ueda, H., Yagi, S., and Kaneko, U. Hydralazine and plasma renin activity. *Arch. Intern. Med.* 122:387, 1968.
29. Sealey, J. E., and Laragh, J. M. Searching out low renin patients: Limitations of some commonly used methods. *Am. J. Med.* 55:303, 1973.
30. Biglieri, E. G., Stockigt, J. R., and Schambelan, M. A preliminary evaluation for primary aldosteronism. *Arch. Intern. Med.* 126:1004, 1970.
31. Brown, J. J., et al. Comparison of surgery and prolonged spironolactone therapy in patients with hypertension, aldosterone excess, and low plasma renin. *Br. Med. J.* 2:729, 1972.

32. George, J. M., et al. The syndrome of primary aldosteronism. *Am. J. Med.* 48:343, 1970.
33. Espiner, E. A., et al. Effect of saline infusions on aldosterone secretion and electrolyte excretion in normal subjects and patients with primary aldosteronism. *N. Engl. J. Med.* 277:1, 1967.
34. Christlieb, A. R., et al. The pattern of electrolyte excretion of normal and hypertensive subjects before and after saline infusions. A simple electrolyte formula for the diagnosis of primary aldosteronism. *Am. J. Cardiol.* 27:595, 1971.
35. Spark, R. F., and Melby, J. C. Aldosteronism in hypertension. The spironolactone response test. *Ann. Intern. Med.* 69:685, 1968.
36. Aitchison, J., et al. Quadric analysis in the preoperative distinction between patients with and without adrenocortical tumors in hypertension with aldosterone excess and low plasma renin. *Am. Heart J.* 82:660, 1971.
37. Nicols, G. L., et al. Percutaneous adrenal venography. *Ann. Intern. Med.* 76:899, 1972.
38. Conn, J. W., et al. Photoscanning of Tumors in Primary Aldosteronism. In Genest, J., and Koiw, E. (Eds.), *Hypertension '72.* Springer, Berlin, Heidelberg, New York, 1972. Pp. 299–312.
39. Horton, R., and Finck, E. Diagnosis and localization in primary aldosteronism. *Ann. Intern. Med.* 76:885, 1972.
40. Brown, J. J., et al. Apparently isolated excess deoxycorticosterone in hypertension. *Lancet* 2:243, 1972.
41. Melby, J. C., et al. 18-Hydroxy-11-deoxycorticosterone (18-OH-DOC) Secretion in Experimental and Human Hypertension. In Genest, J., and Kiow, E. (Eds.), *Hypertension '72.* Springer, Berlin, Heidelberg, New York, 1972.
42. Genest, J., et al. Plasma Progesterone Levels and 18-Hydroxy-deoxycorticosterone Secretion Rate in Benign Essential Hypertension in Humans. In Genest, J., and Kiow, E. (Eds.), *Hypertension '72.* Springer, Berlin, Heidelberg, New York, 1972.
43. Williams, G. H., et al. Abnormal responsiveness of the renin aldosterone system to acute stimulation in patients with essential hypertension. *Ann. Intern. Med.* 72:317, 1970.
44. Bühler, F. R., et al. Plasma aldosterone-renin interrelationships in various forms of essential hypertension. *Am. J. Cardiol.* 32:554, 1973.
45. Carey, R. M., et al. The syndrome of essential hypertension and suppressed plasma renin activity. Normalization of blood pressure with spironolactone. *Arch. Intern. Med.* 130:849, 1972.
46. Douglas, J. G., Hollifield, J. W., and Liddle, G. W. Treatment of low renin essential hypertension. Comparison of spironolac-

tone and a hydrochlorothiazide triamterene combination. *J. A. M. A.* 227:518, 1974.

47. Biglieri, E. G., and Forsham, P. H. Studies on the expanded extracellular fluid and the responses to various stimuli in primary aldosteronism. *Am. J. Med.* 30:564, 1961.
48. Conn, J. W., Rovner, D. R., and Cohn, E. L. Licorice-induced pseudo-aldosteronism. *J. A. M. A.* 205:492, 1968.
49. Christlieb, A. R., et al. Renin: A risk factor for cardiovascular disease? *Ann. Intern. Med.* 81:7, 1974.
50. Stroobandt, R., Fagard, R., and Amery, A. K. P. C. Are patients with essential hypertension and low renin protected against stroke and heart attack? *Am. Heart J.* 86:781, 1973.
51. Gulati, S. C., et al. The occurrence of vascular complications in low renin hypertension. *Ann. Intern. Med.* 78:828, 1973.
52. Doyle, A. E., et al. Plasma renin levels and vascular complications in hypertension. *Br. Med. J.* 2:206, 1973.
53. Genest, J., et al. Renin in hypertension: How important as a risk factor? *Can. Med. Assoc. J.* 109:475, 1973.
54. Freis, E., et al. Veterans Administration Cooperative Study Group on Antihypertensive Agents. I. Results in patients with diastolic blood pressures averaging 115 through 129 mm Hg. *J. A. M. A.* 202:1028, 1967.
55. Freis, E., et al. Veterans Administration Cooperative Study Group on Antihypertensive Agents. II. Results in patients with diastolic blood pressure averaging 90 through 114 mm Hg. *J. A. M. A.* 213:1143, 1970.

4. Clinical Pharmacology of Current and Experimental Drugs

Arthur H. Hayes, Jr.

Although some forms of hypertension have discernible causes (secondary hypertension) that may be amenable to definitive, corrective therapy, as in the case of surgical extirpation of a pheochromocytoma or an aldosterone-secreting tumor, most, perhaps 90 percent, of hypertensive patients are treated with drugs either exclusively and for a lifetime or transiently in conjunction with other modalities. These patients may conveniently be divided into five groups.

The first and by far the largest group consists of those with essential, or primary, hypertension, in whom no specific etiology is apparent. Almost without exception, this type of patient requires drug therapy indefinitely, although it should be noted that all essential hypertension is not uniform in severity nor has the same characteristics. Hence, one may encounter elevated blood pressure with increased peripheral vascular resistance, or with expanded plasma volume, or even with supranormal heart rates and cardiac output. Such distinguishing features may suggest the choice of certain drugs and the avoidance of others.

A second group comprises those with a correctable cause of hypertension, such as pheochromocytoma and elevated circulating catecholamines or renal artery stenosis with markedly elevated peripheral renin activity, in whom specific pharmacologic therapy has been shown to contribute significantly to the preparation for surgery and to overall management.

Related to this group are patients with a diagnosed cause of hypertension, but for whom experience has demonstrated that definitive procedures are rarely, if ever, corrective. Thus, reliance must be placed on pharmacologic measures. Examples include long-standing renal artery stenosis or primary hyperaldosteronism arising from hyperplastic rather than adenomatous adrenal cortical tissue. Here, consideration of the particular features of the syndrome is helpful in designing and evaluating an antihypertensive drug program.

An all-too-common setting for hypertension is concomitant disease in the cardiovascular or other organ systems. These additional problems may actually be caused by the elevated blood pressure, as when left ventricular cardiac failure results; they may, like chronic intrinsic renal disease with impaired function, affect an organ that is being damaged further by the hypertension; and they may be unrelated in these respects, as in the case of asthma or gout. Yet each of these situations makes special demands on the therapist, not only with regard to the consequences of poor or desultory control of the blood pressure, but also in the limitations that may be placed on the choice of drugs because of magnified or special adverse reactions.

Finally, there is "hypertensive crisis," in which the magnitude and progression of the blood pressure elevation pose such an imminent and serious threat to the cardiovascular and central nervous systems that if rapid and adequate therapy is not instituted, disastrous consequences will result. Here, special pharmacologic attributes, including potency, speed of action, and freedom from complicating side effects, are required if therapy is to be adequate and even lifesaving.

Thus, the basis for treatment of most patients with hypertension lies in the use of one or more drugs that have antihypertensive action. Currently, a number of such agents are available or being investigated that have different and often complex, multiple pharmacologic actions and interactions. They do not "cure" hypertension even when a cause is known, but rather reduce the elevated blood pressure level, since it is this phenomenon that we know is associated with increased morbidity and mortality and is susceptible to alteration by drug therapy. The manner in which drugs achieve this result varies and, as we have seen, may consist in a reversal or amelioration of a specific pathologic process, such as reducing increased peripheral vascular resistance by lowering abnormally high renin activity, even though the cause of the uncontrolled renin elaboration is not reversed. The same relatively specific approach is utilized when diuretics, including aldosterone antagonists, are used to reduce blood pressure by contracting the expanded plasma volume seen with unregulated aldosterone production. More frequently, however, the action of the drugs employed is less specific with respect to a particular abnormality and may even involve interference with normal function, as in the blockade of normal sympathetic nervous system activity. In either case, antihypertensive drugs can be expected to alter the homeostatic balance that has resulted from the intrusion of pathologic changes. Since the hypertensive process is a multifactorial and a dynamic one—Irvine Page [1] termed it a mosaic—involving the cardiovascular, nervous, endocrine, renal, and other systems, the changes produced by drugs will lead to often complex compensations elsewhere.

Moreover, all those with hypertension, whatever its nature and degree, do not respond to or tolerate the same drug doses and regimens. Therapy must allow for normal variation and responsiveness to both desired and unwanted drug effects because of individual differences in absorption, metabolism, excretion, and drug sensitivity. Thus, the rational use of antihypertensive agents requires pharmacologic competence, not only to tailor therapy for maximum specificity, but also to interpret correctly the observed effects or lack of them and manipulate the drug or drug combination accordingly.

This does not imply that every patient must undergo an extensive diagnostic evaluation before any drug program can be instituted or modified, for *indeed the vast majority can be effectively and safely treated with a single or a simple combination of drugs,* carefully prescribed and conscientiously monitored. It does mean, however, that if such a pharmacologic awareness guides the physician's choice of drugs and dose regimens, he often will be able to achieve successful control in terms of maximum efficacy and minimal adverse effects more quickly and with greater confidence than without this awareness. All the more will he be in a position to manage maximally complicated and difficult patients for whom "standard" regimens are inappropriate or unsuccessful.

Table 4-1. Representative Antihypertensive Drugs

Type	Generic Name	Trade Name
Diuretics		
Thiazide and related compounds	Chlorothiazide	Diuril
	Hydrochlorothiazide	HydroDIURIL; Esidrix; Oretic
	Chlorthalidone	Hygroton
Loop agents	Furosemide	Lasix
	Ethacrynic acid	Edecrin
Potassium sparing diuretics	Spironolactone	Aldactone
	Triamterene	Dyrenium
Direct vasodilators	Hydralazine	Apresoline
	Minoxidil	
	Diazoxide	Hyperstat
	Sodium nitroprusside	Nipride
Sympathoplegic agents		
Ganglionic-blocking drugs	Pentolinium	Ansolysen
	Mecamylamine	Inversine
	Trimethaphan	Arfonad
Rauwolfia compounds	Whole root	Raudixin
	Reserpine	Serpasil; Sandril; Reserpoid
Peripheral inhibitors	Guanethidine	Ismelin
	Methyldopa	Aldomet
	Pargyline	Eutonyl
Centrally acting compounds	Clonidine	Catapres
Receptor blockers		
Beta blockers	Propranolol	Inderal
	Practolol	
Alpha blockers	Phentolamine	Regitine
	Phenoxybenzamine	Dibenzyline
Miscellaneous agents		
Prostaglandins		

One last general point concerns the problem of patient compliance, which looms so large in this area. Even the ideal regimen is of no value to the patient and gives little satisfaction to the physician if it is not followed. Special problems in long-term care are presented in treating usually asymptomatic patients who are little aware of, or unconvinced of, the risk of their hypertension with drugs that are often expensive in a complicated regimen that may cause unpleasant, embarrassing, and even dangerous side effects. An adequate understanding of the pharmacology of the various drugs can often aid the clinician in assessing, preventing, and solving compliance difficulties. Such an approach also allows, when appropriate, the correct use of fixed drug combinations whose otherwise indiscriminate and even careless prescription based on convenience alone may thwart the therapeutic goal and prove inadvertently harmful.

Therefore, a review of the pharmacologic profiles of the drugs in our antihypertensive armamentarium is appropriate and necessary to any discussion of a practical approach to hypertension (see Chap. 5).

All the drugs currently available or undergoing clinical evaluation for the treatment of hypertension fall into one of four classes (Table 4-1).

Diuretics

Diuretic agents can reduce blood pressure by promoting the excretion of sodium and water, thereby contracting plasma volume. To the extent that excess fluid accumulation underlies elevated blood pressure or aggravates it, as in the case of associated congestive heart failure, this action is significant and helpful. Both the thiazide type (e.g., chlorothiazide, hydrochlorothiazide) and the so-called loop agents (e.g., furosemide) are probably equally effective in appropriate doses, although there have been a few reports suggesting each type as somewhat more effective than the other [2, 3]. One situation in which a loop diuretic is to be preferred is in the presence of severely impaired renal function (creatinine clearance less than 20 ml per minute). In this situation the thiazides are ineffective, and a loop agent that does not further depress glomerular filtration rate should be used. However, any diuretic should be used with caution, if at all, in certain patients with severe renal impairment, the so-called salt losers, in whom salt and water balance may pose special problems.

Spironolactone, an aldosterone antagonist, although generally less potent in terms of maximum effect than the other diuretics, is especially effective when the salt and water retention is secondary to elevated levels of aldosterone and perhaps other mineralocorticoids. However, the substantial cost to the patient for this drug militates against its indiscriminate substitution for other diuretics, which should be tried first in the absence of an indication for aldosterone antagonism.

Although the natriuretic and diuretic actions of these compounds certainly are important to their antihypertensive effect, there is now direct and indirect evidence implicating at least one other mechanism. Some hypertensive patients with initially normal plasma volumes respond to diuretics with both a diminution in plasma volume and a fall in blood pressure. However, the former is often transient and returns to control levels under therapy without a concomitant rise in blood pressure. It has been suggested that this is the result of a direct vasodilating action that, while relatively mild, is often significant. This theory is further supported by the observation that diazoxide, chemically a thiazide, is a powerful vasodilator and yet promotes retention of salt and water. In practical terms, therefore, diuretics should always be tried initially, even in the absence of demonstrable fluid accumulation, unless particular circumstances indicate alternate therapy first.

As many as one-third of all those with mild hypertension will respond to a diuretic alone. But many with more severe or complicated forms of the diasease will not and thus will require additional therapy. Since all nondiuretic antihypertensive agents cause a secondary retention of salt and water that mitigates their effectiveness, a diuretic, even if insufficiently effective alone, should form part of the total drug regimen. Such inclusion will prevent most cases of "pseudoresistance" to other antihypertensive agents and even permit fewer to be used and in smaller doses.

The loop diuretic furosemide promotes a rapid diuresis when administered by the intravenous route; it is also available in a parenteral form. Given intravenously, it has proved especially useful in the edematous patient in whom fluid overload is a contributing factor and in conjunction with parenteral antihypertensives in managing hypertensive emergencies. In these situations, close monitoring of water and electrolyte balance is mandatory.

Side Effects

Fortunately, the use of diuretic agents is not associated with a high incidence of adverse reactions, although in certain circumstances such reactions may be distressing and even serious. The thiazide and loop agents may produce (1) hypokalemia, (2) hyperuricemia, (3) hyperglycemia, and, less commonly, (4) hypercalcemia. Of these, hypokalemia occurs most frequently, but is usually mild, rarely symptomatic, and seldom necessitates discontinuation of therapy. The serum potassium level should be checked before beginning one of these kaliuretic drugs; then, in the absence of specific symptoms or alterations in other therapy, it should be monitored approximately every four to six months. Attention to potassium balance deserves emphasis in the patient with intrinsic heart disease, especially if he is taking a cardiac glycoside, for here the risk of developing cardiac arrhythmias even at relatively lesser degrees of hypokalemia is well documented. Prevention of hypokalemia can usually be accomplished by a high potassium dietary intake in the vast majority of patients (see Chap. 5).

HYPOKALEMIA. When excessive potassium loss is troublesome, a number of corrective measures are available. Occasionally, intermittent diuretic dosage (e.g., alternate-day therapy or therapy five days a week) may maintain potassium economy without impairing antihypertensive efficacy. The judicious inclusion of potassium-rich foods in the diet may be helpful, but the inconvenience and cost of sufficient replacement by this means alone usually renders it impractical. A number of forms of potassium supplements are marketed; however, in adequate dosage, their patient acceptability varies widely. Sometimes, choice of preparation, or mixture with more palatable substances makes this an inexpensive and safe approach to the problem. Too often, however, such remedies are not well tolerated, with a consequent potentially serious lack of compliance. When potassium supplementation is employed for replacement therapy, it probably should be in the form of potassium chloride, since the hypokalemia induced by chronic diuretic administration frequently is accompanied by a hypochloremic alkalosis, and only this salt will remedy the deficit correctly.

When hypokalemia cannot be treated by, or does not respond to, supplementary therapy, the electrolyte imbalance may be corrected by addition of one of the potassium sparing diuretics, spironolactone or triamterene. Both these drugs, which are chemically distinct, act by decreasing the amount of potassium secreted in exchange for sodium in the distal tubule of the kidney. Spironolactone, as we have seen, is an aldosterone antagonist, but the mechanism of action of triamterene is not completely understood. The latter agent by itself does not have significant nondiuretic mediated antihypertensive action. In moderate doses, spironolactone or triamterene may be combined with a kaliuretic diuretic to maintain a normal serum potassium level, usually with minimal discomfort and minimal deleterious side effects. Spironolactone may produce gynecomastia, and triamterene can cause gastrointestinal upsets. Both should be used with great care in the face of renal impairment, for the azotemic patient taking these drugs is prone to serious, even fatal, hyperkalemia. For the same reason potassium supplements should be avoided when a potassium-sparing diuretic is used to maintain a normal serum potassium level.

HYPERURICEMIA. Clinically significant hyperuricemia rarely develops with chronic diuretic use. However, uric acid levels should be obtained before treatment and monitored regularly, if infrequently. In the patient with a history of gout or in whom gout develops, treatment with allopurinol or probenecid will usually allow continuation of the diuretic without recurrent symptoms. An attack of acute gouty arthritis should be managed by appropriate therapy.

HYPERGLYCEMIA. Although instances of acute hyperglycemia have been reported shortly after initiation of a diuretic medication, this is extremely uncommon. Even in the diabetic patient, disturbances in carbohydrate metabolism are seldom of such magnitude to require cessation of therapy. Adjusting diet or hypoglycemic drug dosage may be all that is needed for adequate, safe control. This effect of diuretic therapy is rare but when noted should prompt evaluation of the patient's parathyroid function. Spironolactone may be substituted as a diuretic.

OTHER SIDE EFFECTS. Hearing loss has been reported with both furosemide and ethacrynic acid but apparently is permanent only after the latter [4]. Even though a number of other side effects, among which are blood dyscrasias, gastrointestinal disturbances, and rashes, have been attributed to chronic diuretic usage, they are uncommon and rarely serious. Whether or not the secondary rise in peripheral renin activity that has been described in persons on diuretics is dynamically significant in the hypertensive process remains to be elucidated.

Frequency of administration of oral diuretics depends on the kinetic characteristics of the agent chosen and the total dose prescribed. The long-acting drugs, taken once a day, are more convenient, but electrolyte imbalance may be more troublesome with them. In this connection one seemingly trivial but often annoying problem about which patients may complain is the inconvenience of unaccustomed or more frequent nocturia, especially after an evening dose of a diuretic. When this poses a threat to the regimen, modification of the dose schedule—even prescribing the total daily dose of the short-acting compounds in the morning—may offer an acceptable compromise between optimal control and patient compliance.

Vasodilators

A number of vasodilators have been developed for treating hypertension, but only one oral drug, hydralazine, is now available in this country. The parenteral agents diazoxide and sodium nitroprusside are useful only in hypertensive crises.

Drugs in this group act by directly dilating the arterioles, thereby reducing peripheral vascular resistance and lowering blood pressure. They do not interfere with sympathetic nerve pathways or catecholamine action, and orthostatic hypotension is not seen. As has been mentioned, they promote salt and water retention in effective doses and consequently should always be used in conjunction with a diuretic.

Since these agents do not block sympathetic function, the stimulating action of the carotid sinus reflex induced by the fall in blood pressure may be accompanied by heightened reflex sympathetic activity. This is manifested by increased heart rate, often with palpitations, and elevated cardiac output, resulting in augmented cardiac work and oxygen utilization. While merely annoying to most, it may assume significant proportions in those with heart failure or coronary insufficiency. Indeed, anginal attacks may be precipitated, and frank myocardial infarction has been reported. While use of a diuretic may reduce the tachycardia, wide experience has shown that such effects are most effectively minimized or prevented by the addition of a sympathetic-blocking drug to the regimen. A rauwolfia compound, methyldopa, and guanethidine have all been used with varying degrees of success. As we shall see, the sympathetic blockade they produce is not cardiospecific and may be accompanied by undersirable sympathoplegic actions. Recently, studies conducted in a number of centers have produced convincing data that the beta-adrenergic blocking compound propranolol inhibits this reflex cardiac stimulation without altering normal alpha-sympathetic function, which affects peripheral vascular beds, the gastrointestinal tract, or male reproductive function. This beta blocker also may reduce the secondary rise in peripheral renin activity that has been observed with direct-acting vasodilators and is perhaps mediated by beta-sympathetic pathways. The clinical significance of this phenomenon is not known.

Thus, a regimen consisting of a diuretic, a vasodilator, and a beta blocker, which capitalizes on the actions and advantageous interactions of the component drugs, has grown in popularity for treating patients with all degrees of hypertension including the most severe, even malignant, hypertension [5].

Hydralazine

Hydralazine is a relatively potent antihypertensive agent in its own right and, when given with a diuretic and perhaps a sympathetic-blocking drug, is a most effective one. Its ability to maintain or even increase renal blood flow while lowering blood pressure adds to its value in patients with renal failure. Hydralazine in therapeutic doses is generally well tolerated. However, in addition to salt and water retention and augmented reflex cardiac activity, both of which are usually controllable, it may cause headache, fever, nausea, vomiting and a lupus-like syndrome. This last is most frequent with doses in excess of 200–300 mg daily, and when it occurs, alternate therapy must be substituted. A parenteral form of hydralazine is available for more rapid blood pressure reduction or when oral medication is not feasible.

Optimal doses for an individual patient can usually be attained by using general guidelines and then titrating against depressor response and adverse reactions. The clinician may encounter an unexpected response with respect to dose in the form of lack of efficacy or unanticipated toxicity. While there are many bases for differing sensitivities to the drug, there is now evidence that in some patients sensitivity may be due to genetically determined differences in the rate of hydralazine metabolism [6]. Determination of an individual's rate of drug acetylation, which is the relevant pathway here, is possible in some laboratories and may be helpful in a particularly difficult management problem.

Minoxidil

While hydralazine is the only oral vasodilator on the American market today, other pharmacologically similar agents are under intensive laboratory and clinical investigation. Most prominent among these is minoxidil, and reports of its efficacy in even the most intractable hypertension are very enthusiastic [7]. This compound resembles hydralazine in many respects but appears to have the advantages of greater inherent potency or maximum depressor effect and a longer duration of action—over 24 hours compared with approximately 4–6 hours. In combination with an appropriate diuretic and a beta blocker, it may prove to be as effective as any antihypertensive now known. The hirsutism it can produce may limit its usefulness in women.

Diazoxide

Within the past two years, two parenteral vasodilators, diazoxide and sodium nitroprusside, have been introduced for the rapid control of severely elevated blood pressure, as seen in hypertensive crisis. Diazoxide chemically akin to chlorothiazide, dilates peripheral arterioles, increases cardiac output, and maintains renal blood flow. A maximum fall in blood pressure is usually attained in 5–15 minutes, with a slow rise over the next 2–18 hours. Approximately 15–20 percent of those treated show a minimal response or none at all. It is quickly and almost completely bound to plasma proteins and therefore must be given within 15 seconds to be highly effective. As previously indicated, it provokes salt and water retention and should usually be accompanied by the parenteral diuretic furosemide. Its hyperglycemic potential, which has even prompted its trial in hypoglycemic states, is not usually a significant problem with short-term use in hypertensive emergencies, even in diabetic patients. The nausea, vomiting, fever, flushing, and sweating that may be seen after diazoxide seldom proscribe it when its use is necessary. The side effects of the drug, however, may assume clinical importance when it is given repeatedly or frequently over a number of days rather than switching the patient to oral medications.

Sodium Nitroprusside

Sodium nitroprusside is undoubtedly the fastest and most potent hypotensive agent known and is now available in a stable, lyophilized preparation. When given by constant intravenous infusion, it causes a prompt fall in arterial blood pressure that is dose-dependent, even to subnormal levels. Therefore, continuous monitoring is requisite to safe administration. Its evanescent action allows precise and almost immediate control of blood pressure in most situations with a prompt rise in pressure when the infusion is stopped. A failure to respond to this agent is almost unknown, and it may be used primarily or in those patients who do not respond to diazoxide. Cardiac output is often improved in the presence of heart failure but is otherwise unaffected. Sodium and water retention may occur, suggesting the use of a diuretic, but the moderate reflex tachycardia sometimes seen is usually clinically insignificant. Nausea, retching, vomiting, sweating, twitching, and apprehension have all been described, especially early in the course of treatment, but are seldom more than annoying. One of the major metabolites of sodium nitroprusside is the thiocyanate ion; this may accumulate, especially in the patient with reduced renal function, leading to excitement, confusion, and, rarely, a psychotic state. If infusion must be continued for longer than 72 hours, which is a rare circumstance, blood thiocyanate concentrations should be determined and the infusion stopped if levels exceed 10–12 mg per 100 ml. A detailed discussion of these agents is presented in Chapter 6.

Sympathoplegic Agents

Ganglionic-Blocking Drugs: Mecamylamine and Pentolinium

For many years drugs that block the autonomic ganglia, both sympathetic and parasympathetic, were the mainstay of antihypertensive therapy. Their hypotensive action results chiefly from a fall in cardiac output secondary to a dilatation of the venous bed and a decrease in venous return to the heart, although they also dilate arterioles, causing a fall in peripheral vascular resistance. While they are potent agents, their general use is severely limited because their action is nonspecific, resulting in frequent, annoying, and even serious side effects [8]. Blurred vision, anhydrosis, dry mouth, urinary retention, constipation, and impotence are common in antihypertensive doses, with consequent problems in patient compliance. The significant postural hypotension they produce is hazardous in those with coronary or cerebrovascular insufficiency. Evenness of control may be difficult, since many of these drugs are poorly and irregularly absorbed after oral administration. Their use—always with a diuretic to prevent the anticipated salt and water retention—should be reserved for the rare patient with severe and intractable hypertension who does not respond to or tolerate any of the other regimens now available.

TRIMETHAPHAN. One ganglionic-blocking agent, trimethaphan, has been employed successfully in the management of hypertensive crisis. Given by continuous intravenous infusion, its action develops within 5–10 minutes, and the infusion may then be titrated against the blood pressure response. However, there may be a lag of several minutes between changes in dose and the response produced, and thus the fine control that sodium nitroprusside affords is not usually possible. If the depressor response is greater than desired, a pressor substance such as norepinephrine may have to be used, even though the trimethaphan has been stopped. Since these two compounds work at different sites (at arteriolar receptors and autonomic ganglia, respectively), the pharmacologic antagonism involved is less than desirable and is often difficult to manipulate effectively and safely. Trimethaphan use in hypertensive emergencies should be limited to cases in which the rapidly acting parenteral vasodilators are unavailable, ineffective, or not tolerated.

Rauwolfia Compounds

Rauwolfia serpentina, or Indian snakeroot, has been employed for many centuries in the treatment of mental disturbances and hypertension. During the last few decades the whole root and a number of extracts from the plant have been used extensively to control blood pressure of mild and moderate degree. In fact, in a number of now classic studies that demonstrated the salutary effect of reducing elevated arterial blood pressure such compounds were used [9, 10]. However, the recent advent of more potent and more specific agents that are better tolerated has caused a decline in the use of the rauwolfia alkaloids.

These agents, including the popular reserpine, act to lower blood pressure by interfering with the normal re-uptake of norepinephrine in the peripheral and central sympathetic neurons, thus causing a depletion of this catecholamine in the neuronal granule storage sites. Probably the more important site of action is peripheral, where loss of sympathetic tone results in a fall in heart rate, diminished cardiac output, and, less important, a fall in peripheral arteriolar resistance. All these effects are more pronounced when sympathetic tone is initially elavated. Renin elaboration may also decline due to the sympathetic blocking activity. After oral administration, the antihypertensive action is slow to develop and slow to wane when the drug is withdrawn after long-term usage. Parenteral reserpine is faster and has been employed in acute hypertensive problems.

The rauwolfia alkaloids' general interference with the function of sympathetic and perhaps other biogenic amines, especially in the central nervous system, is certainly related to the lassitude, lethargy, and sedation that is so common with these agents. Severe depression, even to a psychotic degree, has been described and is a serious drawback to widespread and long-term use of these drugs. These mental aberrations are especially troublesome when treating a patient with hypertensive encephalopathy, since the sedative effects of the drug may mask clinical appreciation of changes in the patient's sensorium. In addition, aggravation of peptic ulcer disease and uncomfortable nasal stuffiness may be seen. The recently reported association between reserpine use and breast cancer is disquieting, but its significance has not been established [11].

If one of these compounds is used to treat mild hypertension, it should be with a diuretic and always with careful surveillance of mental status.

Peripheral Inhibitors

GUANETHIDINE. The peripheral inhibitors act by interfering with peripheral sympathetic (adrenergic) function. In the United States, the available compound is guanethidine, which is the most powerful single oral antihypertensive agent known. Its action on the postganglionic sympathetic neuron is complex, but its clinically important effect is an initial interruption of norepinephrine release at the neuroeffector site, followed by a depletion of the catecholamine stores. This results in a fall in heart rate, stroke volume, cardiac output, and, to a lesser extent, peripheral vascular resistance. If pre-drug sympathetic tone is normal, as is the case in many hypertensive persons, a significant reduction in blood pressure may depend on depression of sympathetic function below normal. Renal blood flow may be relatively decreased, and the effect on renin release appears variable. The effector cells are sensitized to catecholamine action, and this heightened sensitivity, even to endogenous circulating amines, may explain some patients' resistance to the drug.

Guanethidine is taken into the adrenergic nerve receptor, its site of action, by an active transport mechanism. This "pump" is inhibited by amphetamines and the tricyclic antidepressants (e.g., imipramine and amitriptyline), and hence concomitant administration of these drugs will antagonize the hypotensive effect.

After guanethidine, blood pressure reduction may be moderate in the supine position but very dramatic in the erect position, due to the marked reduction in the vasoconstrictive response to posture. Thus, smooth control of blood pressure may be difficult. The orthostatic hypotension that should be expected with this drug necessitates adjusting drug dosage for upright blood pressure levels, since postural hypotensive episodes may be alarming and dangerous. Patients should be warned about this possibility and its greater likelihood with exercise or rapid assumption of the standing position. Because of the possibility of abrupt falls in blood pressure, care should always be taken when guanethidine is used in those with coronary or cerebrovascular insufficiency. This effect of guanethidine also explains the relation of its depressor response to fluid balance such that an increase in intravascular volume blunts the blood pressure fall and contraction enhances it. Since secondary salt and water retention occur, judicious use of a diuretic is necessary for optimal action.

Only available in oral form, guanethidine is poorly absorbed from the gastrointestinal tract and does not enter the central nervous system. Several days are required for the development of the full effect of an initial or incremental dose, and, because of its catecholamine-depleting action after long-term use, there is a delay in the reduction of its effects when doses are lessened. This sluggishness in appearance and disappearance of effects requires relatively less frequent (every four to six days) changes in dosage if careful regulation and avoidance of sudden, marked hypotension are to be achieved. Because its metabolism is slow, single daily administration is sufficient. It has been suggested that another agent besides a diuretic be used with guanethidine, not only to reduce the dose necessary but also to smooth out the diurnal variation in blood pressure (lowest in the morning, highest in the evening) seen with large doses [12].

Besides the often marked and disabling orthostatic hypotension seen with guanethidine, the adverse effects most often encountered are diarrhea and failure of ejaculation. Any of these may be so inconvenient or incapacitating that patients will not take the drug or will do so only intermittently and irregularly. The serious consequences of such poor compliance, which often occurs in those with severe hypertension, are well known to physicians who have managed patients on this drug.

BETHANIDINE. Bethanidine is a close relative of guanethidine. It is used in Europe and elsewhere but is not licensed in the United States. Its spectrum of action parallels that of guanethidine, although diarrhea is apparently less common. Its shorter duration of action (8–12 hours) makes dosage adjustment easier, but at the cost of the convenience of a single daily dose.

DEBRISOQUIN. Debrisoquin is another peripheral sympathetic blocking drug that is currently being investigated in this country. The various reports on its use suggest that it is a moderately potent antihypertensive agent, causing a greater fall in blood pressure in the standing than in the supine position. It has some monoamine oxidase–inhibiting properties and, like guanethidine, when given intravenously, may produce an initial pressor response.

ALPHA-METHYLDOPA. Alpha-methyldopa is moderately effective in reducing elevated blood pressure, but its antihypertensive mechanism of action is unclear. Since it is a close congenor of dopa, it has been thought to substitute for this natural precursor of norepinephrine in biosynthetic pathways, resulting in the production of alpha-methylnorepinephrine. This substance then replaces norepinephrine in sympathetic nerve storage granules and, when released by nerve stimulation, results in a diminished vasoconstrictive response. This "false transmitter" phenomenon has been postulated for both peripheral and central sympathetic sites. However, arguments based on experimental observations have called this mechanism into question, and the matter remains unsettled [13].

Regardless of the mechanisms and sites involved, methyldopa is known to reduce peripheral resistance without lowering heart rate or compromising cardiac output. Reflex tachycardia does not occur and may be prevented or reduced when produced by a vasodilating agent. Renal blood flow and glomerular filtration rate are maintained and may even be augmented, making it a highly useful agent in the patient with renal impairment. Although the data are somewhat conflicting, elevated renin activity, whether primary or the result of therapy, may be diminished [14].

Blood pressure reduction may be greater in the standing than in the lying position, but significant orthostatic hypotension is less frequent than with guanethidine, unless plasma volume has been acutely and severely contracted. This can occur when dietary intake and gastrointestinal losses are abnormal, especially in patients with reduced renal function and loss of concentrating ability. This agent is generally safe in those with coronary or cerebrovascular insufficiency, since wide swings in blood pressure are unusual. Salt and water retention are seen, and a diuretic should be used simultaneously. Tolerance with long-term administration, requiring increasing doses has been described. Parenteral forms are available when more rapid action is desired.

After oral administration, methyldopa's absorption varies from 25–75 percent, perhaps partly explaining differences in individual response. Traditionally given three or four times a day, the drug in larger doses on a twice-a-day schedule may, if acute toxic symptoms do not occur, afford equal evenness of control with added convenience and, using the new 500-mg tablet, a saving in cost. Although most of the drug is eliminated unchanged in the urine, toxicity that requires large dosage adjustments seldom occurs, even in advanced renal failure. In fact, many with significantly compromised renal function are exquisitely sensitive to the action of this drug, even though blood levels are not proportionately higher. The presence of methyldopa in the urine does interfere with the fluorimetric assay for catecholamines, but not with vanillylmandelic acid (VMA) or metanephrine determination, a consideration in the diagnosis of pheochromocytoma [15].

Chief among the side effects of methyldopa are sedation and lethargy, which in most patients are transient, even with continuation of therapy, although their persistence is sufficiently incapacitating in some to necessitate withdrawal of the drug. Less common are drug fever, sexual dysfunction in males, abnormal liver function test, and jaundice. Methyldopa is contraindicated in patients with hepatic disease and should be used with caution in those with such a history. In as many as 20 percent of those taking the drug, a positive direct Coombs' test reaction will develop, but since hemolytic anemia rarely occurs, this is important only when it makes cross-matching difficult. Periodic hemoglobin determinations are advised with prolonged therapy.

PARGYLINE. Pargyline is a long-acting monoamine oxidase inhibitor whose potent antihypertensive action is poorly understood. Many theories have been advanced to account for its action, which has been attributed to inhibition of enzymes in addition to monoamine oxidase, depression of norepinephrine synthesis, and production of the false neurotransmitter octopamine. Convincing evidence is lacking for these and other hypotheses, although the multiple actions of this compound have been widely explored. In man, pargyline, taken once a day, produces a significant fall in blood pressure with a pronounced postural component. Since it may take up to three weeks for full activity to appear (which wanes slowly after the drug is discontinued), accumulation, with resulting severe and protracted orthostatic hypotension, can only be avoided by careful dosage adjustments and cautious use of other drugs. A diuretic, however, regularly improves the response to pargyline.

An additional problem faced with pargyline is the inadvertent ingestion of tyramine, which, when its monoamine oxidase–dependent metabolism is inhibited, can cause release of the increased norepinephrine stores and dangerous hypertension. Tyramine unfortunately is found in a number of common foods and beverages, including certain cheeses, beers, wines, chicken livers, and pickled herring, and thus the dietary proscriptions necessary for safe therapy may be very restrictive indeed. Methyldopa, guanethidine, antihistaminic agents, sympathomimetic drugs, and other monoamine oxidase inhibitors should not be used with pargyline [12]. Difficulties in dose regulation and the threat of accidental hypertensive reaction have relegated pargyline's role to special circumstances, and it is rarely used.

Centrally Acting Compounds

CLONIDINE. Clonidine, recently approved by the Food and Drug Administration, differs from all the other compounds thus far discussed by displaying a central mode of action. This is believed to be a central alpha-adrenergic stimulation that results in the inhibition of bulbar sympathetic vasoconstrictor and cardioaccelerator centers and thus in a decrease in sympathetic outflow from the brain [16]. Cardiac output falls, especially in the supine position, but this, it is claimed, tends to return to control levels with long-term clonidine administration. A decrease in peripheral resistance persists, but orthostatic hypotension seems to be infrequent and mild. Heart rate is lowered, which, together with a reduction in venous return to the heart, is thought to contribute to the antipressor effect. Renal blood flow is preserved, and, according to some studies, plasma renin activity is reduced.

Clonidine is usually administered twice daily in incremental doses until adequate control is achieved. The addition of a diuretic enhances the response in most patients.

Reported adverse effects are dry mouth, sedation, headache, and constipation. Abrupt cessation of clonidine therapy has lead to a brief but intense rebound hypertension; thus, doses should be tapered if discontinuation of therapy is necessary, and patients should be warned not to stop the drug without advice. Although wide clinical experience with clonidine is still lacking in this country, it is comparable to methyldopa in potency and may prove a valuable addition to the antihypertensive armamentarium.

Receptor Blockers

BETA BLOCKERS. The only beta-adrenergic receptor blocking drug now available in the United States is *propranolol.* Although licensed for use in certain conditions, e.g., cardiac arrhythmias and angina pectoris, it has not been officially approved for the management of hypertension except that associated with pheochromocytoma. However, since the first report of its antihypertensive activity a decade ago, a voluminous and growing literature has emerged describing its multiple and complex actions in the cardiovascular system and its efficacy, or lack of it, in treating various types of hypertension. It is beyond the scope of this discussion to analyze in detail the very provocative theories and often conflicting data surrounding the pharmacology of propranolol and the plethora of beta-blocking drugs that have been developed [17]. There are, however, a number of delineated beta-receptor antagonist actions that are relevant to an understanding of its depressor activity [18].

Propranolol and related compounds block both the chronotropic and inotropic receptors in the heart, with a consequent fall in cardiac rate and contractility. Since many of these agents also block the peripheral beta receptors responsible for vasodilatation, leaving the peripheral alpha receptors that subserve vasoconstriction unopposed, vascular resistance is increased. Thus, an overall fall in blood pressure may be seen when hypertension is largely due to elevated cardiac output, as in the "hyperdynamic heart syndrome." As has been previously suggested, reliance is placed on this mechanism when propranolol is combined with a direct vasodilator, such as hydralazine, to prevent the reflex increase in cardiac activity that often accompanies the use of such a vasodilator alone. The lack of interference with peripheral vasoconstrictor activity explains the relatively infrequent occurrence of orthostatic hypotension when a beta blocker is employed, as compared with its frequency when a less specific sympathoplegic agent such as methyldopa or guanethidine is administered. An even greater selectivity of action is possible with compounds like the experimental drug *practolol,* which inhibits the beta receptors in the heart to a much greater degree than the noncardiac beta receptors, such as those involved in bronchiolar smooth muscle function or certain metabolic pathways. This type of compound may very well prove to be the most effective and least toxic when used with vasodilators. A serious drawback of all these agents is the possible precipitation or aggravation of heart failure. Therefore, before a beta blocker is administered, a patient should be carefully evaluated for this potential liability and then monitored regularly thereafter. A diuretic drug should always be administered when a beta blocker is used.

Considerable evidence has been gathered pointing to a central site of antihypertensive action for these compounds. Propranolol achieves a high concentration in the brain, and sedation may be seen with chronic use. Often, doses much higher than those necessary for peripheral beta-adrenergic blockade, even up to 2–3 gm per day, are required to lower hypertensive blood pressure levels. Whether or to what extent this reflects inhibition of central catecholaminergic pathways is controversial and experimentally challenging.

Last, considerable attention has been directed lately to the reported ability of propranolol to reduce plasma renin activity [19], especially when it is elevated, as often seen in renal artery stenosis or in some patients with essential or malignant hypertension. This is thought by some to result from an antagonism of the renal sympathetic fibers that are one factor in the control of renin release. However, our understanding of this phenomenon and its possible role in the hypotensive action of propranolol and other beta-blocking compounds is incomplete, for not all those whose blood pressure falls in response to propranolol show a simultaneous decrease in renin activity; conversely, in some, renin activity drops but blood pressure in unaffected. Whether or not propranolol enhances the antihypertensive action of a vasodilator or diuretic [20] by inhibiting the reflex increase in renin activity that these drugs have been observed to produce is also unsettled.

Although many questions regarding the mechanisms of action of propranolol and its appropriate use in various antihypertensive situations are currently unanswered, its antihypertensive efficacy in a significant number of patients seems unassailable. Judicious use of propranolol certainly is logical to reduce a pathologically elevated cardiac output and to prevent the untoward reflex cardiac action that may be brought about by direct vasodilators. It also seems a reasonable therapeutic approach to the management of hypertensive patients with a demonstrated or suspected primary elevation of renin levels or with uncorrectable renal vascular lesions. Wider use of propranolol and other beta blockers based on clearly defined mechanisms must await the further elucidation of their manifestly complex pharmacology, as well as the results of careful clinical trials in various pathologic and therapeutic situations.

Propranolol is well absorbed from the gut, and peak blood levels are reached within 2 hours. A hypotensive effect may be seen shortly after initial administration, but maximum response may be delayed, perhaps because of a long-term downward readjustment in peripheral vascular resistance [21]. The biologic half-life of propranolol after oral administration is a few hours, but its effects may linger after blood concentrations have fallen to almost unmeasurable levels; this may reflect the presence of pharmacologically active metabolites, some of which have been identified. Propranolol is commonly administered three or four times a day, but a twice-daily regimen may prove equally successful [22].

The side effects of propranolol, relating mainly to its beta-adrenergic blocking action, are bradycardia, left ventricular failure and diminished cardiac output, bronchospasm (especially important in asthmatic patients), and hypoglycemia in insulin-dependent diabetic patients, probably due to impairment of compensatory mechanisms in glucose metabolism. Sedation, dreams, insomnia, gastrointestinal upset, rashes, and purpura have also been reported.

ALPHA BLOCKERS. Alpha-adrenergic-blocking drugs interfere with sympathetically mediated vasoconstrictive function. *Phentolamine* is poorly and irregularly absorbed after oral administration and displays a brief duration of action. It has direct cardiac and gastrointestinal stimulating properties and may provoke gastric secretion. *Phenoxybenzamine* is a longer-acting compound that is somewhat unpredictably absorbed from the gut. As might be expected from their selective alpha blockade, both can give rise to reflex tachycardia and postural hypotension, the latter especially when hypovolemia is present.

The difficulties attendant on their use has restricted the place of these drugs to the preoperative and intraoperative management of patients with pheochromocytoma, in whom inordinately high levels of circulating catechomamines may lead to excessive and dangerous elevations in blood pressure.

In this condition they should be used in conjunction with propranolol, which will prevent excessive beta-adrenergic stimulation by the catecholamines.

Miscellaneous Agents

In the search for a more fundamental understanding of hypertension and the mechanisms that underlie it, enthusiasm and investigative fervor now center around the physiologic and pharmacologic actions of the *prostaglandins*. A number of these ubiquitous substances have been isolated and have produced very dramatic effects on blood pressure, leading to suggestions that the presence or absence of various types may play a role in renal parenchymal, renoprival, and perhaps other forms of hypertension. Although appraisal of their therapeutic value in treating clinical hypertension is minimal, there are published reports of their ability to lower blood pressure while increasing cardiac output and renal blood flow [23]. These and similar observations, though preliminary and as yet inconclusive, are exciting, and their further investigation may advance significantly our understanding of hypertension, as well as provide direction for the development of new, more selective, and more potent antihypertensive regimens.

Other contributors to this book will discuss in detail the different applications of these drugs in the treatment of various forms of hypertension. This all-too-brief review of their pharmacology is intended to reinforce the principle that an understanding of their dynamic actions and interactions is essential, indeed crucial, to their correct use. Optimal therapy, which comprises maximal efficacy, minimal toxicity, and a high degree of compliance, demands such an understanding of the available drugs. In hypertensive therapy, nothing is more practical.

References

1. Page, I. H. Pathogenesis of arterial hypertension. *J. A. M. A.* 140:451, 1949.
2. Anderson, J., et al. A comparison of the effects of hydrocholorothiazide and furosemide in the treatment of hypertensive patients. *Q. J. Med.* 40:541, 1971.

3. Mroczek, W. J., et al. Large dose furosemide therapy for hypertension. *Am. J. Cardiol.* 33:546, 1974.
4. Cooperman, L. B., and Rubin, I. L. Toxicity of ethacrynic acid and furosemide. *Am. Heart J.* 85:831, 1973.
5. Koch-Weser, J. Correlation of Pathophysiology and Pharmacotherapy in Primary Hypertension. *Am. J. Cardiol.* 32:499, 1973.
6. Koch-Weser, J. Individualization of Antihypertensive Drug Therapy. (Symposium on Individualization of Drug Therapy.) *Med. Clin. N. Am.* 58(5):1027, 1974.
7. Chidsey, C. A. Clinical and pharmacokinetic studies of minoxidil, a new antihypertensive agent. *Clin. Sci. Mol. Med.* 45:1713, 1973.
8. Pickering, G. *Hypertension.* Churchill/Livingstone, Edinburgh, 1974.
9. Freis, E., et al. Veterans Administration Cooperative Study Group on Antihypertensive Agents. Effects of treatment on morbidity in hypertension. I. Results in patients with diastolic blood pressures averaging 115 through 129 mm Hg. *J. A. M. A.* 202:1028, 1967.
10. Freis, E., et al. Veterans Administration Cooperative Study Group on Antihypertensive Agents. Effects of treatment on morbidity in hypertension. II. Results in patients with diastolic blood pressures averaging 90 through 114 mm Hg. *J. A. M. A.* 213:1143, 1970.
11. Report from the Boston Collaborative Drug Surveillance Program: Reserpine and breast cancer. *Lancet* 2:7882, 1974.
12. Gifford, R. W., Jr. *Hypertension: A Practical Guide to Medical Management.* In *Hypertension Handbook.* Merck Sharp & Dohme, West Point, Pa., 1974. P. 83.
13. Nickerson, M. Drugs Inhibiting Adrenergic Nerves and Structures Innervated by Them. In Goodman, L., and Gilman, A. (Eds.), *The Pharmacological Basis of Therapeutics.* Macmillan, New York, 1970. P. 549.
14. Weidmann, P., et al. Plasma renin and blood pressure during treatment with methyldopa. *Am. J. Cardiol.* 34:671, 1974.
15. Gifford, R. W., Jr., and Tween, D. C. Spurious elevation of urinary catecholamines during therapy with alpha-methyldopa. *J. A. M. A.* 182:493, 1962.
16. Kobinger, W. Pharmacologic Basis of the Cardiovascular Actions of Clonidine. In Onesti, G., Kim, K. E., and Moyer, J. H. (Eds.), *Hypertension: Mechanisms and Management.* Grune & Stratton, New York, 1973. P. 376.
17. Harrison, D. C. (Ed.). *Circulatory Effects and Clinical Uses of Beta-adrenergic Blocking Drugs.* Excerpta Medica, Amsterdam, 1971, P. 113.
18. Kaplan, N. M. *Clinical Hypertension.* Medcom Press, New York, 1973.

19. Bühler, F. R., et al. The Antihypertensive Action of Propranolol. In Laragh, J. H. (Ed.), *Hypertension Manual: Mechanisms, Methods, Management.* Yorke Medical Books, New York, 1974. P. 873.
20. Bravo, E. L., et al. Beta-adrenergic blockade in diuretic-treated patients with essential hypertension. *N. Engl. J. Med.* 292:66, 1975.
21. Tarazi, R. C., and Dustan, H. P. Beta-adrenergic blockade in hypertension: Practical and theoretical implication of long-term hemodynamic variation. *Am. J. Cardiol.* 29:633, 1972.
22. Berglund, G., et al. Propranolol given twice daily in hypertension. *Acta Med. Scand.* 194:513, 1973.
23. Hornych, A., et al. Renal and cardiovascular effect of prostaglandin A_2 in hypertensive patients. *Eur. J. Clin. Invest.* 3:391, 1973.

5. Management of Essential Hypertension

Marvin Moser

I would like to outline what I believe to be a practical method of treatment of the hypertensive patient—one that the practicing physician can follow with good results. I shall concentrate on the management of mild to moderately severe hypertension. The treatment of renal failure with hypertension and hypertensive encephalopathy will be discussed in Chapter 6.

General Guidelines

In Chapter 1 Dr. Stamler discusses high blood pressure as a risk factor and stresses the fact that even a single recording of elevated blood pressure in a young person is of some significance. Significant hypertension will be discovered in a great many people with transiently elevated blood pressures if they are followed for a long enough period of time. Frohlich et al. [1] have demonstrated increased cardiac output and decreased or normal peripheral resistance in these patients and have clearly pointed out that hemodynamically they are different from others in the same age group who do not have wide swings of blood pressure. One of the ideas we must all relinquish is that if someone's blood pressure is elevated when he is nervous, it is of no significance. There are abundant data to show that it *is* of importance in prognosis.

As an example, almost everyone is nervous or anxious during an army physical examination. Why do only a small percentage of the examinees have an elevated blood pressure? Many of these people will demonstrate signs of an overactive sympathetic nervous system, or an inability to metabolize salt properly, or both, and they are potentially hypertensive [2]. A single high (casual) blood pressure recording therefore should not be ignored. All of us demonstrate a marked diurnal fluctuation in blood pressure, with a slowly rising level from early morning to late afternoon. Most of us have a rise in blood pressure during periods of stress. When these diurnal swings or peaks become excessive, they are of significance! Casual pressures have been well correlated with the future development of target-organ involvement (see Chap. 1).

Does this mean that everyone who appears in a physician's office or clinic with a blood pressure of 140–150/90 mm Hg or more need be treated. Not necessarily. It does mean, however, that more attention must be paid to the so-called early neurogenic labile hypertensive (see Table 5-1).

A blood pressure of 140–150/90 mm Hg in any patient under 40 years of age should be a cause for concern. The patient should be advised to return in three to six months to have his pressure checked again. If it is the same, he should be seen in another six months to a year; if it has risen, he should be evaluated and then treated. If, however, the patient smokes, is black, or has additional cardiovascular risk factors—such as a family history of hypertension or stroke, obesity, diabetes or a high blood cholesterol level—he should be placed on therapy sooner than the patient without other cardiovascular risk factors. A patient who presents with a diastolic pressure of

Table 5-1. Treatment Guidelines

Blood Pressure Level (mm Hg)[a]	Response
140/90	Cause for concern, further evaluation, continued observation
90–104 diastolic	Drug treatment probably required
90–104 diastolic, plus other risk factors	Treatment clearly indicated
105 diastolic and above	Drug treatment required on basis of blood pressure alone

[a] Based on at least two or three readings, except in patients with initial diastolic pressures of 110 mm Hg or above, in which case one reading is adequate to establish the need for therapy.

between 90 and 104 mm Hg and other definite risk factors should be treated, especially if blood pressure is elevated on two readings taken over a reasonable period of time. Although long-term data on this group are not clear with regard to increased survival or decreased morbidity, they are highly suggestive that treatment of this group, even before target-organ involvement occurs, is beneficial. If a patient is seen with a diastolic pressure of 105 or 110 mm Hg, he need not be told to come back in a month or two to have his pressure checked again. This is a patient who requires therapy.

Older people present a somewhat different problem. We have all seen patients of 55 years or older with systolic pressures of 180–200 mm Hg and diastolic pressures of 80–90 mm Hg who have been hypertensive for many years and who apparently have done well. Despite this, these patients are at increased risk, with a decreased survival [3]. If their blood pressure can be lowered without producing significant side effects, it should be lowered. Patients 65 years of age and over with elevated blood pressure should also be treated. Obviously, potent drugs that make the patient sick should be avoided. *The risk of treatment must be balanced against the prognosis if untreated.*

The Problem of Systolic Blood Pressure

For years medical texts ignored the problem of systolic blood pressure elevation and advised physicians that this was a phenomenon secondary to atherosclerosis. Treatment was rarely advised. Several other studies [4], as well as the Framingham data [3, 5], have clearly established that the incidence of coronary artery disease and stroke is closely related to elevations of systolic pressure as well as to diastolic levels. Lowering of systolic blood pressure is therefore indicated.

Diagnostic Procedures

Assuming a definite recording of the diastolic pressure of 105–110 mm Hg on one visit or pressures of 140–150/90 mm Hg or more on several visits, what should happen to these patients? First of all, an effort should be made to rule out secondary causes of hypertension clinically, without hospitalization and without complicated studies. This can be done in the vast majority of patients after a careful history and physical examination. If indeed "the extensive work-up is an outmoded fad," what should be done (see Table 5-2) [6]?

The *history* alone can rule out most cases of *pheochromocytoma*. We spend many hours in medical school learning about pheochromocytoma and become very excited about it because it is a very dramatic entity. The vast majority of patients with pheochromocytoma have symptoms; the majority with essential hypertension do not. Therefore, when confronted with the hypertensive patient with definite symptoms, especially sweating, the possibility of pheochromocytoma must be considered. In a patient with no symptoms, the odds of a pheochromocytoma are minimal, and probably no further work-up is necessary. However, if in the course of treatment the patient does not respond appropriately to therapy, treatment can always be stopped and studies such as urinary determinations of vanillylmandelic acid and catecholamines or metanephrines carried out.

An obese patient rarely has a pheochromocytoma. Yes, there are patients with this entity who are obese (we recently followed a 28-year-old patient who was 5 feet 4 inches tall and

Table 5-2. Simple Office or Clinic Studies for Evaluation of Hypertensive Patient

Study	Rules Out	Establishes
History	Most cases of pheochromocytoma Some cases of hyperaldosteronism	
Physical examination	Coarctation of aorta Most cases of Cushing's disease	Severity of hypertension
Urine examination	Parenchymal-renal disease of any significance	
Blood urea nitrogen	Renal failure	
Blood potassium	Most cases of hyperaldosteronism	
Electrocardiogram		Target-organ involvement

weighed 240 pounds who had a pheochromocytoma), but the vast majority of such patients are not obese. Thus, for all intents and purposes, an obese patient need not be studied. Here again, if an inappropriate or poor response to therapy is noted, the tests can always be ordered.

Many patients with clinically significant *aldosterone excess* will have symptoms, including weakness, muscle cramps, polyuria, and polydipsia. Many with clinically significant hyperaldosteronism will be women in the 25–45 age group. These clues should help to select some patients for further study.

Physical examination should rule out coarctation of the aorta; the physical appearance of the patient should in most instances rule out or confirm Cushing's disease. Physical examination should also help to establish the severity of the hypertension. A prominent aortic second sound or an S-4 gallop suggests significant disease.

A clinical finding of interest is the presence of an abdominal bruit. This can be detected by listening to the right and to the left, an inch or two above the umbilicus. Unlike the murmur of an aortic plaque lesion or a lesion in the mesenteric arteries due to arteriosclerosis, this murmur is holosystolic, with a short diastolic component, and is high-pitched (Fig. 5-1). It is suggestive evidence of a renovascular lesion, especially fibromuscular dysplasia, and is an important clinical clue (Table 5-2).

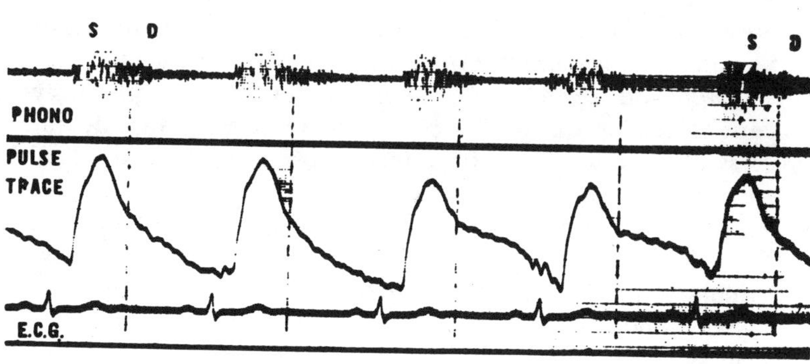

FIG. 5-1. Phonocardiogram of abdominal bruit in renovascular hypertension. (From Moser and Goldman [11].)

What Tests Are Necessary?

A simple urine examination should rule out or establish the presence of renal parenchymal disease in the vast majority of patients with hypertension. Patients with essential hypertension and diastolic blood pressures of under 120–130 mm Hg rarely have proteinuria. A finding of proteinuria in a patient with a diastolic pressure of under 130 mm Hg is therefore significant and strongly suggests the presence of renal parenchymal disease. In a few cases, renal parenchymal disease can exist with elevated blood pressure without proteinuria, but these cases are uncommon.

In patients with diastolic pressures over 130 mm Hg, however, formed elements, as well as proteinuria, may be seen in the urine. In most cases, a negative urinary protein test rules out chronic glomerulonephritis, chronic pyelonephritis, or other parenchymal renal diseases as a cause of the hypertension. A blood urea nitrogen test is a simple way of ruling out or establishing the presence of renal failure.

An *electrocardiogram* is a simple, easy way of determining how much cardiac involvement is present.

Urinary electrolytes need not be done routinely. A *serum potassium test* will rule out most cases of hyperaldosteronism secondary to adrenal adenomas. Urinary electrolyte tests frequently are ordered when a patient is hospitalized, but will rarely give any important hints concerning etiology or treatment possibilities. The urine is collected as a 24-hour specimen, and urinary electrolytes are evaluated without knowing the previous 24-hour sodium and potassium intake. The results are recorded on the chart but rarely influence management.

Intravenous pyelography should be done in all hypertensive patients under the age of 25, in patients with rapidly progressive hypertension, with a history of an injury to the flank, with an abdominal bruit, or in those with resistant hypertension in the older age groups. However, it most certainly need not be done routinely. Since most patients with renovascular hypertension will respond to medical management anyway, and since the risk is high in the older age group and results of surgery often poor, it is usually unnecessary to study these groups of patients for renovascular disease [6].

Arteriography should only be done when the results of a

timed intravenous pyelogram suggest it, or occasionally in young patients with significant hypertension, despite a normal intravenous pyelogram.

The question of determining renin levels, or aldosterone levels, or both has come into prominence in recent years. The excellent work of Conn et al. [7], Gunnells et al. [8], Koch-Weser [9], and Bühler et al. [10] has demonstrated that about 25 percent of patients with essential hypertension have low renin, about 25 percent have high renin, and the rest have normal renins (Fig. 5-2). These investigators have suggested that a more intelligent approach would be to determine the patient's renin levels prior to therapy. While a determination of renin levels may sometimes be of value, the tests need not be done routinely in hypertensive patients, since treatment response will often demonstrate the patient's category, and in

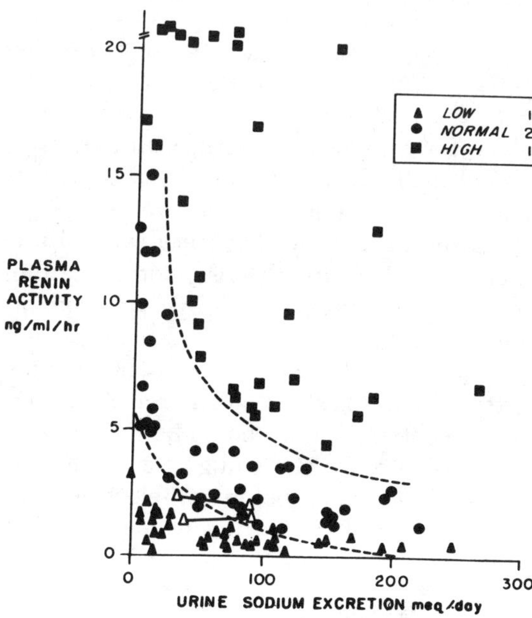

FIG. 5-2. Plasma renin measurements in 51 patients with essential hypertension; 16 patients with low renin, 21 with normal renin, and 14 with high renin are represented, with results related to different sodium excretion rates. (From Bühler, F. R., et al. [10].)

most patients the expenditure of time and money for this test is unnecessary. It is best to start the patient on therapy that he will accept and not to divert him or his physician by doing elaborate and expensive diagnostic work-ups when they can be avoided.

Other Recommended Procedures

A work-up recommended by the Inter-Society Commission for Heart Disease Resources (Table 5-3) includes the following:

Table 5-3. Routine Laboratory and Roentgenographic Examinations Recommended for Evaluation of Hypertension

Hemogram	Blood glucose (preferably 2 hr postprandial)
Routine urinalysis	BUN and/or serum creatinine
Serum potassium	Roentgenogram of chest
Serum cholesterol and triglycerides (for patients $<$ 65 yrs of age)	Electrocardiogram

Adapted from Inter-Society Commission for Heart Disease Resources. *Circulation* 44: A263, 1971.

A hemogram, checking for a high hematocrit; a urinalysis to rule out renal parenchymal disease in most cases; serum potassium determination, which, for all intents and purposes, rules out hyperaldosteronism. Serum cholesterol and triglyceride are listed here only because this is another cardiovascular risk factor, and in the treatment of hypertension, attempts to treat other risk factors of heart disease should certainly be made. (Correction of hypertension alone may not prevent coronary artery disease if other factors remain uncorrected.) A blood glucose determination should be done for the same reason. A blood urea nitrogen test will give an indication of kidney failure, and, as mentioned before, an electrocardiogram will determine the degree of cardiac involvement.

Why Patients Discontinue Treatment

The overall approach to the patient should be directed toward inducing him to accept treatment. We are all told that patient compliance is extremely poor. In some clinics, between 40 and 80 percent of the patients drop out of treatment within a year or two, and many physicians would be surprised if they reviewed their own records of hypertensive patients to find how many have stopped treatment or never returned. Is it always the patient's fault? Before we discuss specific treatment, it is important to consider why patients stop therapy and how, by spending just a few moments with the patient before treatment is begun, we might gain his acceptance of therapy.

Ignorance of Risks in Hypertension

Patients generally stop treatment, first, because they are *unaware of the risk* they face in untreated hypertension. It is not a good idea to tell a patient bluntly that if he does not take his medicine, or that if he continues to have high blood pressure, he will have a stroke, a heart attack, or go into kidney failure. There are ways of conveying this information without producing a panic reaction. We use the booklet *How You Can Help Your Doctor Treat Your High Blood Pressure,* which is now distributed by the American Heart Association. It explains what blood pressure is, what abnormal pressure is, and what some of the risks of untreated blood pressure are; the booklet is reproduced in Appendix 1 of this chapter. It also explains therapy in some detail. We do not frighten the patient unless he is very seriously ill and refuses to continue therapy. It may then be necessary to talk about strokes and kidney failure. We stress that continuous treatment will prevent many of the complications that often occur in patients with high blood pressure.

Lack of Symptoms

Second, the patient may stop treatment because he has no symptoms. It is always easier to treat someone with joint pain, chest pain, or a high fever than someone with asymptomatic high blood pressure. Taking a few moments to explain this problem to the patient during the initial visit or on subsequent visits often converts a poor follow-up result to a good one. This is not a time-consuming procedure.

Follow-up Problems

Third, the patient with high blood pressure is often worried that he will have to visit a physician or clinic frequently for treatment and that visits will be expensive and continue for the rest of his life. Thus, he is reluctant to start on a treatment program. On the other hand, some physicians do not urge patients with high blood pressure to come back at all, and others ask such patients to return at frequent weekly or monthly intervals. Neither method has been successful in treating large numbers of patients. A program that *has* proved to be effective includes visits every three to four weeks during the first few months of treatment or until blood pressure is controlled [11]. If diastolic levels are initially 120 mm Hg or higher, the frequency of visits may have to be increased. It should be explained to the patient that after blood pressure is controlled, he might have to be checked only three or four times a year. (This apparent neglect has not altered good long-term results.) It must be explained to the patient that this is a lifelong treatment program, that drugs will control but not cure high blood pressure.

Expense

Fourth, the cost of therapy can be considerable if patients are on multiple drugs. Fortunately, the vast majority of patients will respond to treatment with thiazides or chlorthalidone, with or without rauwolfia serpentina. Here, the cost may be no more than 10–15 cents a day. In cases where spironolactone (4 pills, 100 mg, a day), or large doses of propranolol (6–8 pills, 240–320 mg, a day) or both and/or adequate doses of alpha-methyldopa (4 pills, 2 gm, a day) are used in addition to diuretic drugs, the cost of therapy may be over a dollar a day. This may represent a real financial burden to the patient. These factors must be kept in mind if the physician wishes to maintain a high level of therapy acceptance.

Side Effects

Fifth, the patient may cease taking medication because of side effects. It is important to stress that if any side effects occur, drugs can be changed or dosage altered. More than 60 percent of patients experience no side effects, *even when potent drugs are used.* It is also important to stress that the patient's life-style need not be changed either by his disease or by the therapy. Patients can participate in sports, perform any kind of manual labor, and lead a perfectly normal life if they take their medication and blood pressure is controlled. Any restrictions tend to decrease compliance and contribute to a poor response rate.

Restrictions, If Any

ALCOHOL. Alcohol in moderation need not be ruled out. Smoking is not to be encouraged, although smoking a few cigarettes a day will generally have little effect on blood pressure. Chain smoking, however, will elevate blood pressure as a result of catecholamine release and will result in an increase in heart rate and cardiac work. Patients should be advised to stop smoking—not necessarily to control blood pressure but in an attempt to eliminate another risk factor in cardiovascular disease.

DIET. There is no longer any need for the hypertensive patient on drug therapy to restrict his diet drastically. Although there is good evidence that treatment with a diet containing less than 500 mg of sodium a day will lower blood pressure, the vast majority of patients will not follow such a restricted diet for long periods of time. On the other hand, there is some evidence that a high-salt diet (over 15–20 gm per day) will make blood pressure control difficult despite the use of diuretics [12]. A compromise program works very well. Patients are advised to cut down on their salt intake by eliminating potato chips, pretzels, and other obviously highly salted foods, such as corned beef, or hot dogs. This will usually reduce their salt intake from the average United States intake of about 10 gm per day to about 5 gm. Diuretics are effective at this level of salt intake, and patients will accept this minor level of restriction.

Some investigators have advocated both salt and carbohydrate restriction in the management of hypertension [12a]. A low carbohydrate intake will decrease the amount of salt reabsorbed in the small bowel and will also increase sodium excretion by the kidneys. In some instances, this type of management may reduce the dosage of drugs required for blood pressure control. The patient must discipline himself to follow this type of diet, and many patients are unable to do so. Our experience has demonstrated that the less change in life-style that is imposed on the patient, the better chance of long-term success. (See Appendix 2 at the end of this chapter.)

Compliance and Follow-up

Some studies have demonstrated that in a large number of patients compliance will occur only if there is a careful follow-up in the home. The Baldwin County, Georgia, study demonstrated clearly that when patients were followed up by a nurse or physician's aide visiting them in their home, checking their pressures, and otherwise following them carefully, compliance was much higher than when this type of follow-up was not available (Fig. 5-3). This type of approach is obviously not possible for most physicians, who practice without benefit of public health grants. Obviously, we must attempt to accomplish the same thing by educating and motivating patients to stay on therapy.

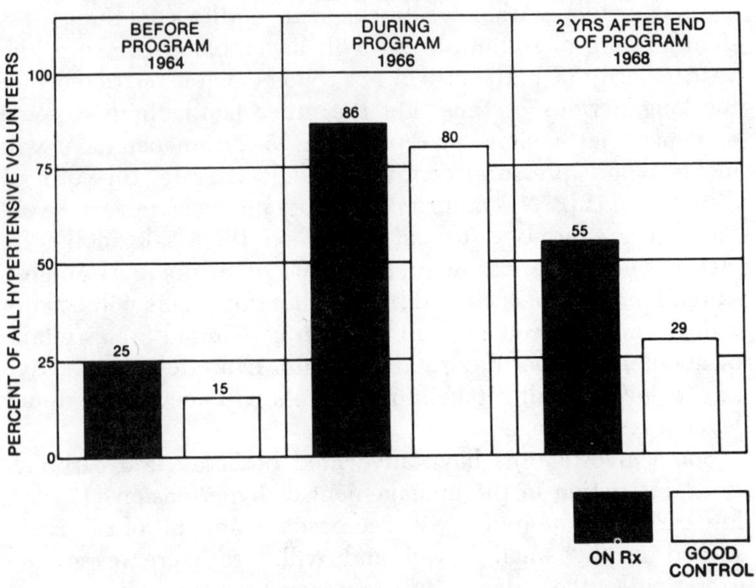

FIG. 5-3. Effects of home follow-up on 88 hypertensive volunteers. Percentage on treatment and good control before, during, and two years after the program. (From Wilber and Barrow [13].)

Home Blood Pressures

Taking blood pressures at home may be helpful in a small percentage of patients who are receiving multiple and potent drugs and who might have an occupation that requires frequent postural changes. It may also be helpful if adjustment of dosage is difficult, especially with guanethidine. In our experience, however, we have not found this procedure necessary in the vast majority of patients. We believe it contributes to anxiety and makes the family and the patient overly conscious of blood pressure. One goal of treatment is to prevent the patient from becoming neurotic about his blood pressure. An attempt should be made to treat him without significantly altering his life-style or his home situation.

However, a 48-year-old dentist whom we have treated for the past 15 years provides a good example of how home blood pressures may be helpful. His occupation required that he stand in one place for many hours a day, and blood pressure control was not achieved until guanethidine dosage was 125 mg per day. Frequent episodes of weakness occurred in the morning during the first few months of therapy as drug dosage was being increased. The patient was instructed to take his own blood pressure several times a day and adjust guanethidine accordingly. After six months a stable dosage was reached, and home readings were discontinued.

Outline of Therapy

In Chapter 4, the actions and side effects of the available antihypertensive drugs are discussed in detail. Table 5-4 reviews the dosage and side effects of commonly used, effective oral drugs that are approved for use in hypertension. I would like to emphasize certain basic points of treatment and outline a simple method of therapy. Many physicians are treating hypertensive patients with drugs but are not achieving good results. There are thousands of patients receiving one or more drugs, who are investing their time, effort, and money in treatment, but whose blood pressures are not being treated to an end point. Treatment *by definition* must be lowering of the blood pressure to normotensive or near normotensive levels, if at all

Table 5–4. Characteristics of Most Commonly Used, Orally Effective Drugs Presently Approved for Use in Hypertension

Drug	Trade Name	Dosage (mg/day)	Side Effects[a]
Diuretics			Serum chemistry abnormalities: $\downarrow$ Potassium, $\uparrow$ Uric acid, $\uparrow$ Urea nitrogen, $\uparrow$ Blood glucose
Chlorothiazide	Diuril	1000	
Hydrochlorothiazide	HydroDIURIL Esidrix	100–150	Leukopenia, anemia, thrombocytopenia
Bendroflumethiazide	Naturetin	10	Skin rashes, purpura, photosensitivity
Methyclothiazide	Enduron	10	Weakness
Polythiazide	Renese	4–8	
Furosemide	Lasix	40–80	Gastrointestinal upsets, pancreatitis
Chlorthalidone	Hygroton	50–100	
Rauwolfia derivatives			Sedation, bradycardia, nasal congestion, nightmares
Reserpine	Serpasil	0.1–0.25	Depression
Whole root	Raudixin	50–100	Activation of gastric ulcer
Alseroxylon fraction	Rauwiloid	2–4	Breast cancer?[c]
Deserpidine	Harmonyl	0.25	
Hydralazine	Apresoline	100–250	Headaches, tachycardia, nausea Increase in angina pectoris Rheumatoid-like syndrome, lupus reaction[b]
Guanethidine	Ismelin	10–150 or more	Weakness, diarrhea, loss of ability to ejaculate Orthostatic hypotension
Methyldopa	Aldomet	500–2500	Drowsiness, depression, edema, impotence Abnormal liver function tests, fever Orthostatic hypotension
Clonidine	Catapres	0.1–0.4 mg	Drowsiness, fatigue

[a] Many side effects are rare, for example, blood dyscrasias and pancreatitis with diuretics.
[b] Rare with doses under 300 mg.
[c] Relationship not proved.

possible. Treatment may include as little as one 50-mg dose of hydrochlorothiazide three or four times a week or as much as 15 to 20 pills and four or five different drugs a day. The blood pressure must be titrated to a satisfactory level.

The best example of drug titration is in the treatment of atrial fibrillation. If a patient had a ventricular rate of 140 beats per minute and was given what was considered to be a "full digitalizing dose" but did not respond, the dosage of digitalis would be increased until the rhythm broke to a regular sinus rhythm, or until the ventricular response rate was under 70, or side effects or abnormal rhythms developed that were suggestive of digitalis toxicity. The same basic therapeutic program should be applied to the treatment of hypertension. Therapy must be increased until a therapeutic end point is achieved or until significant side effects develop. In the more serious cases, some side effects may have to be tolerated if the prognosis, without treatment, is poor.

Step 1

DIURETICS. In a patient without target-organ involvement (grade 1 hypertension), basic therapy consists of an oral diuretic agent. This can be any one of the drugs listed in Chapter 4 (Table 4-1), starting with 50 mg of hydrochlorothiazide and building up to levels of 100 mg per day if the patient does not respond (Table 5-5). In younger patients, and in some older ones, 1 tablet three times a week might be effective. If in several months the response is not adequate, dosage should be increased. Obviously, the higher the initial blood pressure and the more significant the risk factors, the more therapy is needed initially and the more vigorously it is pursued, with more frequent increases in dosage.

Concern on the part of some physicians regarding excess potassium loss with the use of diuretics, especially in elderly patients, often results in withholding adequate treatment. In our experience, however, clinically significant hypokalemia is rare in the vast majority of patients, although serum potassium levels may decrease by approximately 0.5 mEq per liter. The average American diet contains approximately 60–100 mEq

Table 5-5. Ambulatory Medical Therapy of Hypertension

Severity	Drugs of Choice	Additional Prescription If Needed
Grade I, with no organ system involvement		
a. Diastolic BP < 110 mm Hg	1. Oral diuretic 2. Rauwolfia	1. Hydralazine (Apresoline) 2. Propranolol (Inderal)
b. Diastolic BP > 110 mm Hg	1 and 2 above plus Hydralazine	1. Alpha-methyldopa (Aldomet) or 2. Guanethidine (Ismelin) 3. Propranolol
Grade II or *III,* with heart, kidney or brain involvement Diastolic BP's usually > 110 mm Hg	1. Oral diuretic 2. Rauwolfia 3. Guanethidine	1. Hydralazine 2. Alpha-methyldopa 3. Additional diuretics 4. Propranolol

of potassium daily.* Since the minimum daily potassium requirement is only about one-half to one-third of this, or 20–40 mEq K^+ per day, a significant deficiency is not produced in the majority of patients while they are taking diuretics. The extra daily intake of 20–25 mEq of potassium that probably is necessary to prevent hypokalemia in these patients is usually provided by the normal relatively high potassium dietary intake. However, if a deficiency occurs (serum K < 3.2 mEq per liter), it may require an extra 40–60 mEq per day of potassium to correct it and maintain normal levels. In these cases, the use of potassium supplements or potassium-sparing agents may be necessary.

Appendix 2 includes an instruction sheet that we have used to inform our patients about the potassium content of food and to list some of the more commonly used potassium supplements.

DRUG COMBINATIONS. In some patients with tachycardia or signs of increased cardiac output, palpitations, or nervousness, a

* One mEq of potassium is equal to 39 mg K^+.

combination of a rauwolfia preparation and an oral diuretic, or propranolol and a diuretic, might be indicated. This type of combination results in catecholamine depletion and reduces blood pressure by volume depletion.

Combination therapy is frequently indicated with several of the antihypertensive drugs. It is not a good idea, however, to use a combination tablet in which one drug is extremely potent, since dosage titration is frequently difficult. Such combinations as rauwolfia serpentina and bendroflumethiazide (Rauzide); reserpine, hydralazine, and hydrochlorthiazide (Ser-Ap-Bs); hydrochlorthiazide and reserpine (Hydropres); chlorthalidone and reserpine (Regroton) and others are useful. The number of required pills and the cost are reduced, and the fewer pills the patient takes, the less seriously ill he thinks he is. Obviously, the problem of treatment would be much simpler if we had one pill that combined three or four different ingredients, was effective in most cases, and was long-acting. Unfortunately, such a medication is not available.

Some physicians are loath to use the *rauwolfia* drugs because depression is a possible side effect. This should be watched for, and if a patient begins to have insomnia, dreams, or nightmares, the drug should be stopped.*

Step II

HYDRALAZINE. If a combination of an oral diuretic with a rauwolfia drug or propranolol does not work after a suitable period of time, the addition of hydralazine in gradually increasing doses, up to a maximum of between 200 and 250 mg per day, is indicated; the increases in the dose of hydralazine can be provided by giving the patient 25 mg twice a day for three or four days and then 50 mg twice or three times a day. This is continued for four to six weeks, until the patient's next visit. Hypotensive overshoots are rare from hydralazine (Apresoline), and the initial side effects of headaches or palpitations generally will not result if the patient is pretreated with rauwolfia serpentina or propranolol. If these symptoms

* Recent reports linking the long-term use of rauwolfia drugs with a possible increase in the incidence of breast cancer in older women require confirmation.

do occur, they are probably secondary to an excessive amount of histamine (since hydralazine blocks histaminase) and can be countered by an antihistaminic. They usually disappear within a few weeks. The so-called hydralazine syndrome is extremely rare when doses are kept below 250–300 mg per day and should not be a deterrent to using hydralazine in treatment. Dosage is then increased to 50 mg four times a day if normal blood pressure has not been achieved. The use of Ser-Ap-Es, a drug combining a rauwolfia compound, hydralazine, and a diuretic may be useful.

Patients with diastolic blood pressures of 110 mg Hg or higher or with evidence of target-organ involvement, such as left ventricular hypertrophy, usually require the use of oral diuretics plus rauwolfia plus hydralazine or other drugs for good results. The diuretic and rauwolfia should probably be started together and the patient seen within two to three weeks. If no response is obtained, the addition of hydralazine is indicated.

ALPHA-METHYLDOPA. If, after one or two months, blood pressure control is not achieved, the addition of alpha-methyldopa is indicated. Alpha-methyldopa is gradually increased from 250 mg three times a day to doses of up to 2 gm per a day. One of the major problems with this drug is that it is frequently underused or overused. In the 50 percent of patients who do not respond, it is often continued despite the lack of response. We have collected a large number of cases in which alpha-methyldopa and a diuretic were given, and the physician was secure in the knowledge that he was "treating the patient," but blood pressures are uncontrolled. This is not the fault of the drug, but in the way that it is given. If a response is not obtained with a combination of a diuretic and alpha-methyldopa with hydralazine, the addition or substitution of one of the more potent agents such as guanethidine is indicated.

PROPRANOLOL. Although propranolol (Inderal) has not been approved by the F.D.A. for use in hypertension as yet, there are many cases in which it has been used successfully. We have followed a group of patients in whom propranolol in doses of between 80 and 400 mg per day, combined with a diuretic, has produced good blood pressure responses. The combination of propranolol, a diuretic agent, and hydralazine has been effective in some patients who have not responded to alpha-methyldopa and a diuretic. Unfortunately, because the drug is new, it is being overused. We have observed hypertensive patients who have been treated with propranolol with a poor response and whose therapy was not changed. In these cases, it is important to stop propranolol and try another drug.

Step III: Guanethidine

Patients with more severe disease frequently require a combination of three, four, or even five drugs, and in most cases, the use of guanethidine is necessary. Guanethidine is started in doses of 12.5 mg per day (½ tablet) and increased every three to four days until either a good blood pressure response is obtained or the patient experiences significant side effects. When guanethidine is used, the patient usually must initially be seen every four to five days, but when control is achieved, the patient need be seen only three or four times a year. A major problem with guanethidine is postural hypotension. This generally is less pronounced after several weeks or months of treatment, and most patients adjust to this since the pressure remains low. We have had to stop administration of the drug in several young male patients in whom ejaculatory impotence developed; this, in our experience, is a major problem with the use of guanethidine. However, guanethidine is by far the most potent orally effective drug available and is sometimes the only drug that will produce good results in a difficult case [13a]. The major mistake in therapy is that the dosage of guanethidine is frequently not increased to an end point, i.e., to normal blood pressure in the upright position. We have used as much as 350 mg per day of guanethidine.

In our recent series of some 242 patients followed over an average of 8.9 years, 5 patients were on five drugs and a total of 9 on four drugs simultaneously for long periods of time.

Antihypertensive Drugs and Renin

The effects of antihypertensive drugs on renin were discussed in Chapter 4. I would like to review some of these data and show how the physician, without actually obtaining renin levels on his patients, can use the data in establishing guidelines for treatment.

Certain agents have a definite effect on plasma renin (Table 5-6); for example, the vasodilators, such as hydralazine, and the diuretic drugs increase renin levels [9]. Nonetheless, the diuretic agents are extremely effective in almost all hypertensive patients, including those with low renin (volume-dependent hypertension).

Propranolol, reserpine, alpha-methyldopa, and possibly guanethidine act to lower plasma renin levels. There is a practical way to use this information without complicating the work-up and making it more expensive by obtaining renin levels. If the patient has not responded to medication and is already receiving a diuretic, hydralazine, methyldopa, or guanethidine, the substitution of propranolol for one of the others might be indicated. If a lowering effect on blood pressure is noted, it is possible that the patient had high renin hypertension. Many patients with renal parenchymal hypertension or renovascular hypertension have high renin levels. These patients may therefore be responsive to propranolol.

An illustrative case is that of a 34-year-old woman who had chronic glomerulitis proved by biopsy (Fig. 5-4). Management

Table 5-6. Hemodynamic and Hormonal Effects of Antihypertensive Drugs

Drugs	Cardiac Output	Total Peripheral Resistance	Plasma Volume	Plasma Renin Activity
Diuretics	0, +	−	−	+
Propranolol	−	0, +	0	−
Vasodilators	+[a]	−	+	+
Guanethidine	−	−	+	?
Reserpine	0, −	−	+	−
Methyldopa	0	−	+	−

[a] No increase with sodium nitroprusside.

NOTE: + = increase; − = decrease; 0 = no change.

Adapted from Koch-Weser, J. *Am. J. Cardiol.* 32:499, 1973.

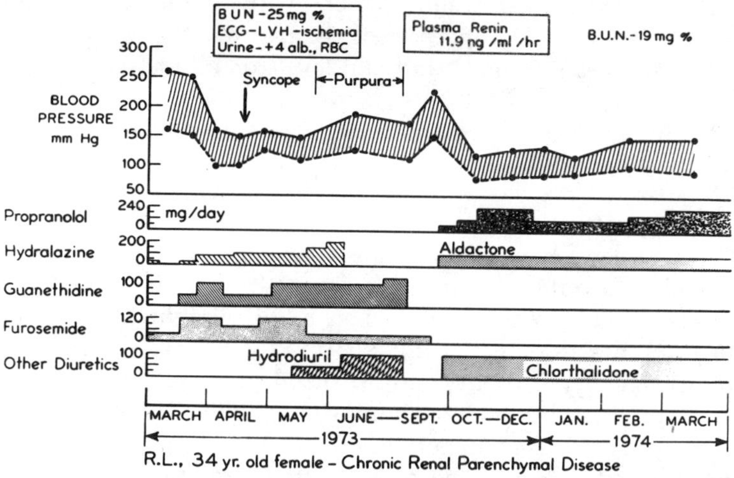

FIG. 5-4. An example of a highly motivated patient with "high-renin" hypertension who persisted in therapy despite its many side effects. In May, 1975, blood pressure was 140/90 mm Hg, and the patient was asymptomatic. (See text for details.)

of her hypertension was extremely difficult. The use of guanethidine controlled her blood pressure but resulted in syncope. The thiazide diuretics caused a purpuric reaction. Finally, propranolol was added to the treatment program, chlorthalidone was substituted for the thiazides, and spironolactane was given because of a persistently low serum potassium. Blood pressure control was quickly achieved and maintained, with few symptoms. Plasma renin levels were elevated (11.9 ng per milliliter per hour) prior to the use of propranolol. This patient demonstrated renal function impairment and extremely high blood pressures. Her prognosis, untreated, based on many studies, was at the most three to five years. Her prognosis is now good, based on our experience with similar patients who have been well controlled over many years.

This patient responded promptly when propranolol was added to a regimen that had included multiple drugs. She was highly motivated and was willing to try many different regimens despite side effects. As a practical matter, propranolol can be used in a resistant patient without obtaining renin levels. Renin is only one part of the treatment spectrum, and it is not necessary to obtain renin levels on all patients.

Long-Term Follow-up

Case Report

An example of how patients can be managed in office practice is well illustrated by the case of a 42-year-old man who, typically, had no symptoms when he was originally seen for an insurance examination in 1953 (Fig. 5-5). He showed left ventricular hypertrophy, and his blood pressure was over 140 mm Hg diastolic and 220 mm Hg systolic. There were no signs of accelerated hypertension, however, and he was not hospitalized or submitted to exhaustive investigative studies. He was placed on varying medications, including 600 mg of hydralazine. However, the "hydralazine syndrome" developed, requiring approximately six weeks on corticosteroid therapy to clear. Following the use of ganglion-blocking agents, which are no longer in general use, and various other medications, his blood pressure was finally controlled when the thiazides became available. He has been followed over the past 18 years, during which he has been on thiazides, with an excellent blood pressure response. His electrocardiogram has changed from one showing left ventricular hypertrophy with both

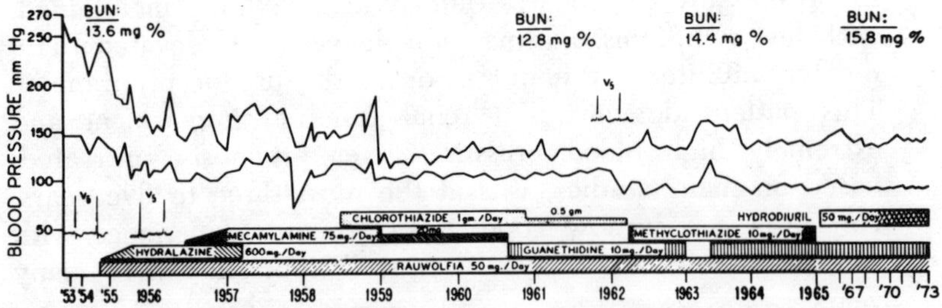

FIG. 5-5. Excellent long-term response to therapy in a 42-year-old man with grade II hypertension. Control was greatly improved after use of diuretics in 1958. In April, 1975, his blood pressure was 135/80 mm Hg, and he was asymptomatic.

voltage and T wave and S–T segment criteria for ischemia to one that is relatively normal. His blood urea nitrogen has remained normal. Although initial control of his blood pressure was not easy, medication was added and changed until a good result was obtained. The patient's motivation has been excellent. He has retired, skis and plays golf regularly, is in excellent health, and is now examined only twice yearly.

In over 35 percent of patients with initial left ventricular hypertrophy followed by us, we have noted the clearing of hypertrophy on electrocardiographic studies. The results in this case are typical of the effects that can be expected from good long-term treatment.

Effects of Long-Term Treatment on Kidney Function

Moyer et al. [14] have shown in many studies that long-term antihypertensive therapy may also be beneficial in terms of improving renal function. The fear of a further decrease in renal function due to a long-term effort to lower blood pressure is obviously unfounded. Figure 5-6 shows that of patients with diastolic blood pressures of under 130 mm Hg, those who were treated had a slight fall in glomerular filtration rate but a lesser fall than those who were untreated. In patients with higher diastolic pressures, those treated had a minimal fall in

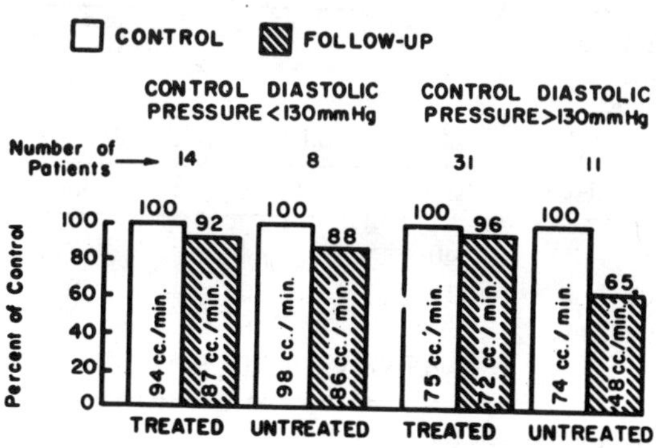

FIG. 5-6. Data on glomerular filtration rate in treated and untreated patients, demonstrating lack of progression of renal impairment in patients on antihypertensive therapy (see text for details). (From Moyer et al. [14].)

glomerular filtration rate, but those not treated had a significant fall. Other investigators have also reported that, despite the initial fall in glomerular filtration rate following the lowering of blood pressure, the long-term results on kidney function have been beneficial.

The treatment of hypertension with complications and the management of malignant hypertension is discussed in Chapter 6.

What Can Be Accomplished by the Simple Practical Approach?

What can a physician expect to achieve in his office or in a clinic if he takes just a few minutes to talk to patients to inform them of their diagnosis, treats them vigorously, and follows them carefully? In a long-term private practice experience with 242 patients over a 19-year period, 85 percent of the patients achieved excellent blood pressure control, defined as blood pressure of 140/90 mm Hg or below (Table 5-7) [15]. These results were obtained regardless of the initial blood pressure.

Table 5-7. Results of Long-Term Treatment of Hypertension[a]

Number of Patients	Pretreatment Diastolic Blood Pressure Level (mm Hg)	Blood Pressure Results		
		Excellent[b]	Fair[b]	Poor[b]
51	115+	40	4	7
128	105–114	112	10	6
63	90–104	54	6	3
Total: 242		206 (85%)	20 (8%)	16 (7%)

[a] Average duration of follow-up was 8.9 years.
[b] Excellent: 140/90 mm Hg or less. Fair: decrease in blood pressure of 20/10 mm Hg or more but not to normotensive levels. Poor: decrease in blood pressure of less than 20/10 mm Hg and not to normotensive levels.
From Moser [15].

Vascular Complications

What kind of complications can the physician expect if he treats hypertensive patients vigorously? Fourteen serious complications have been noted in our series of 242 treated patients. Over 50 percent of all patients had target-organ involvement prior to treatment. As noted, 85 percent showed an excellent blood pressure response. There were seven complications (four myocardial infarctions and three cerebrovascular accidents) in the 206 patients with an excellent blood pressure response. Therapy had not been started in any of these patients until after age 45 or after hypertension had been present for a number of years. In the 36 patients with fair to poor blood pressure response, there were also seven complications (two myocardial infarctions and five cerebrovascular accidents). None of these patients had been started on treatment until they had had hypertension for many years.

There have been no cases of pulmonary edema in controlled patients and no evidence of progressive renal failure in patients who started on therapy with a creatinine level of under 3 mg per 100 ml or a blood urea nitrogen under 40 mg per 100 ml.

Obviously no statistical significance can be assigned to these data since patients were not matched prior to onset of therapy, etc., but the small number of complications in a series of this size over a long period of time is of interest. It will be interesting to follow other studies to judge whether or not earlier treatment might reduce complications even further.

Although the present study cannot be compared with others because there were no matched controls or randomization of patients, it is of interest to compare several series of untreated patients with several series of treated patients as a rough guide (Fig. 5-7). In Bechgaard's [16] series, in a 4- to 11-year follow-up, there was a 25–30 percent mortality. In Palmer's [17] series, there was a 35 percent mortality in 18 years in a mildly severe group of hypertensive patients. The Leichman [18] series, which included moderately severe to severe cases, had a 50 percent mortality in 11 years in the untreated cases. The Veterans Administration study [19], which has been alluded to, shows that therapy resulted in a marked decrease in mortality (from 10 percent to approximately 3 percent over 3.3

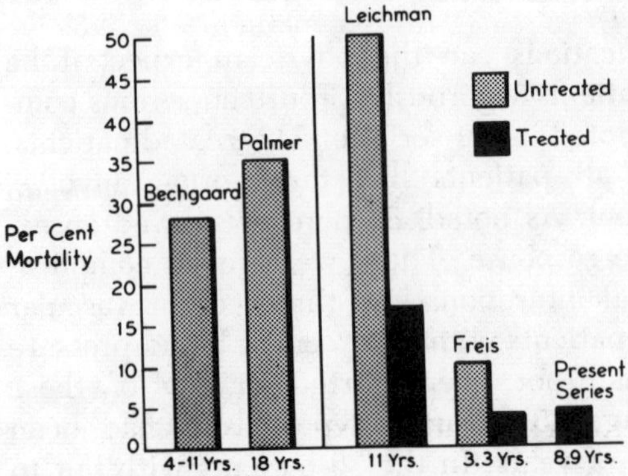

FIG. 5-7. Data comparing different treated and untreated series of hypertensive patients [15–19]. A marked decrease in mortality is noted following treatment.

years) and a sharp decrease in complications: 84 in untreated patients versus 24 in treated patients (Table 5-8). In our own series, over an average of 8.9 years, the mortality rate was 4.5 percent (Table 5-7).

Conclusions

The management of hypertension must be changed from a complicated, expensive program to a simple, practical one if we are to truly alter this serious cardiovascular risk factor. This can be done without sacrificing scientific or academic

Table 5-8. Results of Treatment of Hypertensive Vascular Disease, Veterans Administration Cooperative Study Group on Antihypertensive Agents

Treatment Status	Number of Patients	Blood Pressure Diastolic (mm Hg)	Complications	Deaths	Average Duration of Follow-up
Control	70	115–129	23	4	20 months
Treated	73		2	0	
Control	194	90–114	57	19	3.3 years
Treated	186		14	8	

From Freis et al. *J.A.M.A.*, Dec. 11, 1967, Vol. 202, p. 1028. Copyright 1967 American Medical Association.

curiosity. We are not suggesting two-tier medicine: exhaustive studies for those who can afford it and few studies for those who cannot. We are suggesting a uniform program of studying patients who need to be studied, treating the ones who show elevated blood pressure, whether or not they have target-organ involvement, and treating them to normotensive levels over long periods of time, using some of the methods that have been described to gain better patient compliance.

Recent data appear to indicate that treatment for mild to moderately severe hypertension will reduce strokes, progressive heart failure, and progressive renal failure. The data on myocardial infarction are not so impressive. However, there are no data on patients who were treated early and followed over a long period of time; the patients who have been reported on usually had not been started on treatment for several to many years after hypertension was diagnosed. It appears that complications specifically related to elevated blood pressure, such as ruptured aneurysms and strokes, can be controlled. Simultaneous control of other risk factors, such as blood lipids and cessation of smoking, might be necessary to have a real impact on some of the arteriosclerotic complications.

The patient with hypertension should be able to face the future with optimism. But only by a concerted long-range program can we reverse some of the statistics cited in Chapter 1. Only by a massive physician and lay education effort can we change the mortality tables of insurance companies and keep thousands of people in useful occupations and away from rehabilitation centers. It may be dramatic to treat the end results of hypertension—stroke, kidney failure, or coronary disease—but it should be more rewarding to all of us to prevent the drama from taking place at all.

References

1. Frohlich, E. D., Tarazi, R. C., and Dustan, H. P. Hyperdynamic β-adrenergic circulatory state. *Arch. Intern. Med.* 123:1, 1969.
2. Paffenbarger, R. S., Thorne, M. C., and Wing, A. L. Chronic disease in former college students. *Am. J. Epidemiol.* 88:25, 1968.

3. Kannel, W. B., et al. Epidemiologic assessment of the role of blood pressure in stroke. The Framingham Study. *J. A. M. A.* 214:301, 1970.
4. Gubner, R. S. *Life Expectancy of the Younger Hypertensive—Hypertension—Recent Advances.* Lea & Febiger, Philadelphia, 1961.
5. Dawber, T. R., and Kannel, W. B. Susceptibility to coronary heart disease. *Mod. Concepts Cardiovasc. Dis.* 30:671, 1961.
6. Moser, M. A simplified approach to hypertension. *Am. J. Fam. Pract.* 7:117, 1973.
7. Conn, J. W., et al. Normokalemic primary aldosteronism. *J. A. M. A.* 193:100, 1965.
8. Gunnells, J. C., et al. Plasma renin activity in healthy subjects and patients with hypertension. *Arch. Intern. Med.* 119:232, 1967.
9. Koch-Weser, J. Correlation of pathophysiology and pharmacotherapy in primary hypertension. *Am. J. Cardiol.* 32:499, 1973.
10. Bühler, F. R., et al. Plasma aldosterone-renin interrelationships in various forms of essential hypertension. *Am. J. Cardiol.* 32:554, 1973.
11. Moser, M., and Goldman, A. G. *Hypertensive Vascular Disease.* Lippincott, Philadelphia, 1967.
12. Moser, M. The effect of a high salt diet on the treatment of essential hypertension. In J. H. Moyer, *Hahnemann Symposium on Hypertension.* Saunders, Philadelphia, 1959. P. 512.

12a. Goldman, A. G. Personal communication, 1975.

13. Wilber, J. A., and Barrow, J. G. Reducing elevated blood pressure—Experience found in a community. *Minn. Med.* 52:1303, 1969.

13a. Moser, M. Guanethidine and bethanidine in the management of hypertension. *Am. Heart J.* 77:423, 1969.

14. Moyer, J. H., et al. The vascular status of a heterogeneous group of patients with hypertension with particular emphasis on renal function. *Am. J. Med.* 24:164, 1958.
15. Moser, M. Office management of hypertension. *Am. J. Fam. Pract.* 10:152, 1974.
16. Bechgaard, P. The Natural History of Benign Hypertension. In *Epidemiology of Hypertension.* Grune & Stratton, New York, 1967.
17. Palmer, R. S. Treatment of hypertension. *J. Chronic Dis.* 10:500, 1959.
18. Leichman, A. W. D. Hypertension—Treated and untreated. *Br. Med. J.* 1:5134, 1959.
19. Freis, E., et al. Veterans Administration Cooperative Study Group on Antihypertensive Agents. Effects of treatment on morbidity in hypertension. I. Results in patients with diastolic blood pressures averaging 115 through 129 mm Hg. *J. A. M. A.* 202:1028, 1967.

Appendix 1: How You Can Help Your Doctor Treat Your High Blood Pressure*

Your doctor has just told you that you have high blood pressure (hypertension) and that you need treatment. It is important that you understand a few things about blood pressure in order for you to cooperate as fully as possible with your physician. Hypertension is no longer a disease to be feared; yet you cannot sit back and ignore it. Recent studies have shown that modern treatment is helpful and can prevent many of the complications that occurred in some patients prior to the availability of effective therapy.

What Is High Blood Pressure?

Normally, when a doctor records your blood pressure, he writes down two numbers, an upper one called the systolic pressure and a lower one known as the diastolic pressure.

For example, $\frac{120\text{ (systolic)}}{80\text{ (diastolic)}}$.

The systolic pressure represents that blood pressure in the arteries when the heart is pumping, and the diastolic pressure is the pressure in the arteries at the time the heart is filling with blood for the next beat.

Usually, in any person under the age of 40 a systolic pressure greater than 140–145 is elevated. However, in patients of 60 to 70 years of age a systolic pressure of 150–155 may be within normal limits. When the diastolic pressure is consistently greater than 90–95, the diagnosis of hypertension is justified. This means that even when the heart is at rest the pressure in the arteries is too high and this may lead to blood vessel damage. It is important to remember that blood pressure levels change from minute to minute, with posture, exercise, tension, smoking, and sleeping. Because of these fluctuations, the *trend* of the blood pressure over a period of time (weeks or months) is more important than one isolated measurement.

People who have high blood pressure are not always overanxious, compulsive or tense. Although high blood pressure may run in families, many people with a strong family history of high blood pressure never develop it. High blood pressure affects all ages, but is noted most frequently in persons over 40 years old.

* Adapted from *How You Can Help Your Doctor Treat Your High Blood Pressure* by M. Moser, © 1974, American Heart Association, Inc., reprinted with permission. This booklet, available through local heart associations for patient use, has been extremely helpful in gaining patient cooperation in hypertension therapy.

What Causes High Blood Pressure?

Most people who demonstrate an elevated blood pressure have what is called *essential hypertension,* meaning the cause is unknown. While much research is continuing on this disease, thus far the precise reason for the elevated blood pressure remains to be discovered in over 90 percent of patients—those with essential hypertension.

Other forms of high blood pressure are caused by kidney disease, tumors of a gland near the kidneys, or the narrowing of certain arteries, and may be completely correctable. For example, if high blood pressure is caused by a narrowing of an artery supplying a kidney, repair of this artery will often cure hypertension without further treatment. Most of these abnormalities can be ruled out by a careful history, a physical examination, or a few simple tests. Special tests are occasionally necessary.

How Does Hypertension Develop?

Ordinarily, blood is pumped by the heart through the arteries of the body. After supplying the many organs of the body with much needed oxygen and nutrients, it returns to the heart through veins. Somewhere in between there are small vessels that are able to dilate (become larger) and contract (become smaller) under the influence of certain nerve impulses. If these vessels are wide open, blood can flow through easily, and no increase in the strength of the heartbeat is necessary to force the blood through. If, however, these vessels become narrowed, the heart must pump with a greater pressure to force the blood to flow effectively.

If the blood vessels remain small, and the heart keeps beating forcefully, not only does the heart become strained, but blood vessels may become damaged. Eventually, changes in the vessels supplying blood to the kidneys and the brain may produce changes in these organs. Fortunately, the heart, brain, and kidneys are able to withstand increased pressure for long periods of time. That is the reason why many patients with high blood pressure may go along for years without *any* symptoms or ill effects. However, it has been shown that high blood pressure is one of the most important risk factors in heart attacks, strokes, and kidney failure.

What Can Be Done for High Blood Pressure?

How can you help your blood vessels and vital organs withstand the added burden of hypertension, and how can your doctor help you? Obviously, the strain on your heart can be reduced simply by reducing the demand for blood in various parts of your body. Fatty tissue requires a lot of blood to feed it. Therefore, if you are overweight, the first way to reduce the load is to lose weight. A low-fat or low-cholesterol diet and weight reduction (in addition to blood pressure lowering) may also help delay the onset of arteriosclerosis (hardening of the arteries).

Moderate exercise is not only permitted but should be encouraged. However, avoid overexertion. If you participate in sports, stop playing when you are tired.

The excess fluid that sodium (salt) retains in the body also may put an added burden on the heart. Thus, specific low-sodium diets are also used in treating hypertension. However, the restriction must be drastic (more than just omitting table salt or salt in cooking) if diet *alone* is used, and most patients have found it impractical to continue such restrictions for any length of time. Rigid sodium restriction is probably not necessary in the treatment of high blood pressure since, in most instances, medications called diuretics may be prescribed that help to rid the body of excess sodium. You can keep the sodium content of your diet at a reasonable level by avoiding such salted foods as peanuts, processed foods, salt pork, milk, and milk products and not adding extra salt to other foods.

There is no reason why a person with high blood pressure cannot drink alcohol in moderation. But if you are on a weight reduction diet, remember that alcohol is high in calories. Smoking, another important risk factor of coronary heart disease, should be reduced, or eliminated if possible.

Learning to relax for short periods of time during the working day, at night, and on weekends is, of course, extremely helpful. Also, try to get plenty of sleep since blood pressure is lowest during sleep and rises during waking hours.

What About Treatment with Drugs?

There are many ways to relax or dilate blood vessels. The diuretic agents are usually the cornerstone of most treatment programs. By eliminating excess sodium from the body, these medications are helpful in controlling blood pressure. The most commonly used diuretics are chlorothiazide (Diuril), hydrochlorothiazide (Esidrix, HydroDIURIL, Oretic), bendroflumethiazide (Naturetin), and chlorthalidone (Hygroton). All of these act in a similar manner although there may be differences in duration of action. Your doctor will probably use the one with which he is most familiar.

If diuretic therapy is not effective in bringing blood pressure down to normal levels, your physician may add other drugs to the treatment program. Frequently, a combination tablet containing a diuretic agent and one of the other specific blood-pressure-lowering drugs may be used. This will reduce the number of tablets that you might require each day.

Among the more effective drugs that may be used are rauwolfia derivatives (reserpine), hydralazine (Apresoline), guanethidine (Ismelin), alpha-methyldopa (Aldomet), and propranolol (Inderal). These drugs relax the narrowed blood vessels by direct action on the muscular wall of these vessels or by blocking the nerve supply that causes at least part of the narrowing. The vessels dilate or relax, and blood pressure lowering occurs *only* during the period of time that the drugs are effective. Medication cannot, therefore, be stopped *even after* a satisfactory response has occurred, and in most cases some treatment must be continued indefinitely to produce a continuous good result.

If you are being treated with any or several of these drugs, the dose of the drug or drugs must be carefully regulated, and you must be seen regularly by your doctor—*at least until blood pressure is controlled.* After that, visits may be less frequent.

You are an individual with your own unique medical history, life-style, and reactions. Your physician may have to try several drugs before he finds the one that is best for you—the one that lowers your blood pressure and gives you the least side effects.

What Are Some of the Side Effects of Drugs That Lower Blood Pressure?

Certain nerve impulses that control other functions of the body, in addition to those that control blood pressure, are often blocked by some of the above medications. This influence on other systems sometimes produces side effects. This does not mean that you will always experience a side effect. Most patients have taken these drugs without any problems. But if you do have side effects, the most common ones are the following:

1. *Diuretic drugs* may produce a decrease in the body stores of potassium. Symptoms such as weakness, leg cramps, or tiredness may result. Dietary potassium supplements (such as taking an extra-large glass of orange juice or a banana once or twice daily) while receiving the diuretic will help to prevent a low potassium in most patients. Many doctors prevent potassium loss by administering it in the form of a liquid or a tablet along with the diuretic, especially in patients receiving digitalis for heart disease. Additional drugs such as spironolactone (Aldactone) or triamterene (Dyrenium) might also be prescribed.

Occasionally, gout may be precipitated in susceptible individuals after prolonged treatment with diuretics. Your doctor may prescribe colchicine to control acute attacks and allopurinol (Zyloprim) or probenecid (Benemid) to prevent further attacks.

In patients with diabetes, diuretic drugs may increase the blood sugar level. This can be corrected in most cases by a change in diet, insulin, or oral diabetic drug dosage. Your doctor is well aware of these side effects and will adjust his management accordingly.

2. *Rauwolfia drugs* (reserpine) may produce a stuffy nose, occasional diarrhea, or heartburn. These effects are not severe and no treatment is required other than a dosage adjustment. If nightmares, insomnia, or depression occur (these are rare) your doctor should be informed, and the drug discontinued.

3. *Hydralazine* (Apresoline) may produce headaches, swelling

around the eyes, palpitations, or aches and pains in the joints. Usually, none of these symptoms are severe, and most will disappear after several weeks of treatment. If they persist, your doctor may combat these annoying reactions by prescribing other drugs.

4. *Guanethidine* (Ismelin) may produce some diarrhea. Generally on continued treatment this side effect will become less troublesome. Because this drug reduces blood pressure to a greater degree when the patient is in the upright position, he may experience occasional dizziness, lightheadedness, and feelings of extreme weakness when he gets out of bed in the morning or stands up suddenly. If you note any of these reactions and they persist for longer than a minute or two, it is important to sit down or even lie down and either reduce or omit the next dose of the drug. If symptoms continue, you should contact your doctor.

In the beginning, you may find it helpful to raise the head of the bed a few inches for sleeping, to get out of bed slowly, and not to stand still for more than a few minutes. When you are taking guanethidine, do not remain standing in the hot sun or at a cocktail party if you begin to feel faint or weak. Any of these activities may dilate blood vessels further and cause low blood pressure. Male patients taking the drug may note a form of impotence which is not harmful, but which can be quite annoying. If this symptom persists, your doctor may have to change the drug dosage.

5. *Alpha-methyldopa* (Aldomet) may also produce a greater fall in blood pressure in the upright position and may cause a feeling of weakness or faintness if pressure has been lowered too far. A dosage adjustment will generally eliminate these symptoms. This drug may also cause drowsiness, dryness of the mouth, fever, or anemia.

If you know beforehand about some of the above symptoms and know what to do about them, it will be easier for you to continue with treatment. Your patience will usually be rewarded by a good long-term result.

Some Final Advice

It should be clear that the modern treatment of hypertension may be complicated and may require a great deal of time and care on the part of both the doctor and the patient. It is annoying to take pills and experience side effects when you may have felt fine before treatment. Don't be discouraged if you must continue treatment indefinitely. All of this effort is far less than that required to treat the complications of high blood pressure, if and when they occur. Most cases respond to therapy, and most patients whose blood pressure has been successfully treated live a long and *normal* life.

It should be emphasized that not everyone with hypertension should be treated with drugs listed above. Some people may do just as well on other therapy. Your physician should not be forced to use a certain medication because you have read about its wonderful effect on other people. You could conceivably have a serious side effect from taking a "wonder drug" that wasn't indicated in the first place. Let your doctor decide what, if any, drug to use.

Here is some good advice to help you learn to live with your high blood pressure and to know what to expect from treatment:

1. Don't be frightened by high blood pressure. It can be treated effectively.
2. Do the simple things that your doctor suggests. Simple measures, especially weight reduction and diuretic therapy, often produce good results.
3. Don't rush frantically from one physician to the next, looking for a quick, easy "miracle drug." Stick to one reliable doctor or one good clinic, and follow through with the plan of treatment.
4. If you do find yourself on drug therapy, be patient and don't stop treatment if some annoying side effects occur.
5. Give yourself a chance to adjust to the drug's reaction. It often takes several weeks to do so, but the end results well justify your persistence.

This information is general. Only your doctor can give you precise details and instructions.

Appendix 2

The following dietary instruction sheet has also been helpful to use in gaining patient acceptance of hypertension therapy.

Patient's Dietary Instruction Sheet

Your physician is treating your high blood pressure with a medication called a *diuretic*. This drug increases the amount of salt or sodium that is washed out of your body. Diuretics may also cause a decrease in the body stores of another mineral called *potassium*. Most of the time, an adequate diet will prevent excess potassium loss. In some cases, especially in older people, or when a patient is taking a medicine called *digitalis,* it may be necessary to give extra potassium as a tablet or liquid. This may also be true in patients with kidney disease, or when symptoms of weakness or muscle cramps occur. Kaon, Kaochlor, potassium chloride, K.Ceil, and Slow K are commonly used medications.

The following lists may give you an idea of which foods to eat or stay away from in order to keep your potassium intake high and your salt or sodium intake low.

1. Foods relatively high in potassium but also high in sodium or salt.
   These foods should be avoided, if possible.
   Tomato juice, canned
   Clams, raw
   Sardines
   Lima beans, frozen
   Peas, frozen
   Peas, canned
   Spinach, canned
   Carrots, canned
2. Foods relatively high in potassium and low in sodium.
   Extra amounts of these foods will prevent a potassium deficiency.

Fruits	*Vegetables*
Apples, raw, whole	Asparagus, frozen
Apricots, canned	Beans, white, cooked
Apricots, dried	Beans, snap, green, cooked
Avocado	Brussel sprouts, fresh, frozen
*Banana	Cabbage, shredded
Cantaloupe	Cauliflower, fresh, frozen
Dates, dried, pitted	Corn on the cob
Grapefruit	Lima Beans, fresh, cooked
Nectarine, raw	Peas, green, cooked
Prunes, dried, cooked	Peppers, green, raw
*Raisins, dried, seeded	*Potato, baked
Watermelon	Potato, boiled, no skin
	Radish, red, raw
	Squash, frozen, cooked

Fruit Juices
Apple Juice, fresh, canned
Grapefruit, canned
Prune, canned
*Orange juice, fresh, canned, frozen

* Especially helpful.

6. Management and Prognosis in Complicated Hypertension

Ray W. Gifford, Jr.

The goal of antihypertensive therapy is to prevent the cardiovascular and renal complications, disability, and premature death that characterize the natural history of hypertension. There is now good evidence that the goal is attainable for patients with diastolic blood pressure over 104 mm Hg [1–3], and there is presumptive evidence that patients with lower levels of diastolic blood pressure will also benefit from therapy [2, 3].

Unfortunately, many hypertensive patients are not identified, or treated, or both until complications occur. Since most of the cardiovascular complications of hypertension compromise prognosis with or without hypotensive treatment [4–7], it is unwise to wait until there is evidence of target-organ damage before initiating antihypertensive therapy, as advocated by some physicians in the past. Moreover, the first manifestation of some of the complications of hypertension, such as stroke and myocardial infarction, may be fatal or permanently disabling.

On the other hand, hypotensive therapy should not be withheld once complications have appeared, because there is evidence that reducing blood pressure will improve the prognosis, even though it is not as good as if complications had never occurred [3–5].

The presence of target-organ damage therefore has an important bearing on prognosis and, in many cases, on the choice of antihypertensive drugs and the urgency with which they are administered. Consequently, one of the prime objectives of evaluation of the hypertensive patient is to detect evidence of target-organ disease.

The target organs of hypertension are the brain, the eye, the heart, the kidney, and the peripheral arteries. The hypertensive complications that occur in these organs are listed in Table 6-1. Most authorities classify the complications of hypertension as either atherosclerotic (e.g., cerebral infarction, angina, or myocardial infarction) or "hypertensive" (e.g., hypertensive encephalopathy, cerebral hemorrhage, exudative retinopathy, hypertensive heart disease, and arteriolar nephrosclerosis). In general, antihypertensive therapy has been more effective in preventing the truly hypertensive complications than in preventing the atherosclerotic complications [1–3]. Less is known about the efficacy of antihypertensive therapy in secondary prevention (once complications have already

Table 6-1. Complications of Hypertension

Target Organ	Complications	
	Atherosclerotic[a]	Hypertensive
Brain	Transient ischemic attacks (TIA) Cerebral infarction	Hypertensive encephalopathy Cerebral hemorrhage
Eye	Retinal vascular accidents	Exudative and hemorrhagic retinopathy Papilledema
Heart	Angina pectoris Myocardial infarction Sudden death	Hypertensive heart disease (cardiac hypertrophy, cardiomegaly, ECG-LVH, congestive heart failure)
Kidney	Renal vascular disease[b]	Arteriolar nephrosclerosis (with or without fibrinoid necrosis of arterioles)
Peripheral arteries	Atherosclerotic occlusion of aorta and its branches Intermittent claudication	Dissection of aorta

[a] Complications of atherosclerosis can occur in normotensive individuals, but they tend to be more severe, more frequent, and to occur at an earlier age in hypertensive patients.

[b] Whereas atherosclerotic occlusion of the renal artery can cause hypertension, it may also sometimes be the result of hypertension.

Table 6-2. Response of Some Complications of Hypertension to Antihypertensive Therapy

Complication	Response to Therapy	
	Initial	Tends to Prevent Recurrence
Hypertensive heart disease	Excellent[a]	Yes
Angina pectoris	Good	Yes
Myocardial infarction	?	Yes (?)
Hypertensive encephalopathy	Excellent[a]	Yes
Transient ischemic attacks	Good	Yes
Cerebral infarction	?	Yes
Cerebral hemorrhage	Poor	Yes (?)
Neuroretinopathy	Excellent[a]	Yes
Renal failure		
Serum creatinine 1.5–3.0 mg/100 ml	Good	Yes[b]
Serum creatinine 3.1–8.0 mg/100 ml	Fair	Sometimes[b]
Serum creatinine > 8.0 mg/100 ml	Poor	No[b]

[a] Usually reverses clinical manifestations completely.
[b] Since renal failure is seldom, if ever, reversed, these responses refer to prevention of progression rather than recurrence.

occurred) than in primary prevention. Table 6-2 lists the anticipated responses of some of the complications of hypertension to antihypertensive therapy.

Prognosis in Complicated Hypertension with and without Treatment

Evidence of target-organ damage, irrespective of which organ or organs are involved (Table 6-1) worsens prognosis in treated and untreated hypertensive patients (Table 6-3) [3–7].

Ocular and Renal Complications

Ocular and renal complications coexist so frequently that they will be discussed together.

The presence of exudative retinopathy with papilledema (Keith, Wagener, Barker group 4, or malignant hypertension) is the worst prognostic sign. More than 80 percent of untreated

Table 6-3. Prognosis in Complicated Hypertension, Treated and Untreated

Number of Complications[a]	Percent Mortality (5 years)			
	Men		Women	
	Not Treated	Treated	Not Treated	Treated
None	38.1	14.8	25.7	7.9
One	50.0	31.7	22.6	14.6
Two	100.0	50.0	81.8	23.8

[a] Congestive heart failure angina, stroke, and azotemia.
From Smirk [4].

patients with this manifestation die within the first year [6–9]. Renal involvement, as indicated by proteinuria (more than a trace), or azotemia, or both, is probably the next most unfavorable sign. Often, malignant hypertension and renal insufficiency coexist, and this makes the prognosis even more dismal and definitely limits the effectiveness of treatment.

Antihypertensive therapy unquestionably prolongs life in patients with malignant hypertension [10–16]. Perry [16] has reported that the long-term prognosis for nonazotemic patients with malignant hypertension on adequate medical therapy was actually better than for treated patients with group II hypertension that was complicated by coronary or cerebrovascular disease. The five-year survival for treated patients with malignant hypertension was 60 percent if azotemia was not present, but only 25 percent if azotemia was present [16].

Retinal hemorrhages, exudates, and papilledema disappear when blood pressure is reduced. Permanent loss of vision is uncommon unless there has also been a retinal vascular accident. A retinal vascular accident by itself does not seem to influence prognosis unfavorably, but there is no evidence that effective antihypertensive treatment will prevent or hasten the resolution of this primarily atherosclerotic event.

Cerebral Complications

Transient ischemic attacks (TIA) are often harbingers of a stroke. At least 20 percent of patients with TIA will have a cerebral infarct within five years [17]. It is a clinical impression that reduction of blood pressure usually reduces the frequency of TIA and in some cases completely eliminates it. Whether or not the occurrence of stroke is thereby reduced is unknown.

A history of cerebral infarction compromises prognosis for the untreated hypertensive patient [4, 5]. The magnitude of the stroke seemed to make no difference in Smirk's series [4], but Simpson and Gilchrist [7] reported that only major strokes had an unfavorable influence on prognosis. With one exception [18], there is agreement that antihypertensive treatment for patients who have had one cerebral infarction reduces the frequency of recurrent strokes and prolongs life [19–21]. Marshall's data [19] are summarized in Table 6-4. The Cooperative Study of the National Institute of Neurologic Diseases and Stroke [18] failed to show any significant differences in survival or frequency of recurrent strokes between their placebo and treated groups, but the patients in this study differed from those in the other reports in that they had mild hypertension and 80 percent were black.

Hypertensive encephalopathy and *intracerebral hemorrhage* are medical emergencies. Both conditions are fatal in over 80 percent of untreated patients. Prompt reduction of blood pressure using parenteral agents is associated with complete recovery in nearly all patients with hypertensive encephalopathy,

Table 6-4. Effect of Antipressor Therapy on Prognosis in Patients with Cerebral Infarction (Three-Year Follow-up)

Group	Number of Patients		Number of Nonfatal CVAs	Number of Deaths
	Men	Women		
Treated	18	21	8[a]	4[b]
Untreated	25	17	22	12[c]

[a] In six patients; four had TIA only.
[b] Two died of a cerebrovascular accident (CVA).
[c] Eight died of a CVA.
From Marshall [19].

unless irreversible brain damage has occurred because treatment was delayed. There is no convincing evidence that prompt reduction of blood pressure is beneficial for victims of intracerebral hemorrhage. Some physicians are of the opinion that it is potentially dangerous to reduce blood pressure drastically because of the accompanying vasospasm that is frequently seen on angiograms around the area of hemorrhage. The controversy is largely academic, because an intracerebral hemorrhage is so catastrophic that few patients survive with or without antihypertensive therapy, and those who do are usually severely disabled.

Very little is known about the ultimate fate of patients who have recovered from hypertensive encephalopathy, but Hamilton [22] found that they seemed to be predisposed to the development of cerebrovascular accidents even with antihypertensive therapy. Of 17 patients who recovered from hypertensive encephalopathy and who received long-term antihypertensive therapy, 5 subsequently died from stroke within one to seven years, and 2 others had nonfatal strokes.

Cardiac Complications

Ischemic heart disease. Any of the manifestations of atherosclerotic heart disease (angina pectoris or historical or electrocardiographic evidence of myocardial infarction) worsens the prognosis for the hypertensive patient [6, 23, 24], just as they do for the normotensive patient. Several investigators have observed improvement in angina pectoris when blood pressure is reduced [22, 25, 26]. Except for one study that offers evidence that effective hypotensive therapy prolongs life and reduces the occurrence of myocardial infarctions for hypertensive patients who already have clinical evidence of ischemic heart disease [27], none of the treatment trials has conclusively shown that effective reduction of blood pressure prevents the complications of atherosclerotic heart disease. However, in the Veterans Administration study [1, 2, 3], there were twice as many sudden deaths in the placebo group as in the treatment group (8 versus 4). Atherosclerotic heart disease is the most common cause of death among treated hypertensive patients [2, 28].

HYPERTENSIVE HEART DISEASE. Cardiomegaly by roentgenogram, ECG evidence of left ventricular hypertrophy or strain or both, and left ventricular failure are each and collectively associated with increased mortality in untreated hypertensive patients [4, 6, 7, 23, 29, 30]. From their Framingham experience, Kannel and colleagues [29] have reported that definite electrocardiographic evidence of left ventricular hypertrophy (ECG-LVH) carries a threefold risk that clinically overt coronary heart disease will develop, even after adjustment for the effect of coexisting hypertension. As a matter of fact, the mortality for patients with definite ECG-LVH was similar to that for patients who have survived a myocardial infarction.

Although dyspnea without other manifestations of hypertensive heart disease was not associated with increased mortality [7], overt congestive heart failure was associated with a poor prognosis in the Framingham study [30]. Within five years of onset, 60 percent of men and 40 percent of women died of the manifestations of congestive heart failure.

Fortunately, antihypertensive therapy has been shown to be extremely effective in treating and preventing recurrences of congestive heart failure secondary to hypertensive heart disease [3, 10, 26]. Whereas left ventricular failure was once the most common cause of death among untreated hypertensive patients, it is now among the least common causes of death in those who are treated [28]. When it does occur, it is almost invariably associated with poor control of blood pressure or severe renal failure. Reduction of blood pressure in patients with hypertensive heart disease not only eliminates the symptoms, but often leads to a reduction in cardiac size on the roentgenogram (Fig. 6-1) [10, 14, 15] and improvement or reversal of electrocardiographic abnormalities (Fig. 6-2) [10, 14, 15, 25, 26, 31, 32].

In spite of these salutary effects of antihypertensive therapy on the manifestations of hypertensive heart disease, it is unlikely that the long-term prognosis for treated patients who have had clinical evidence of hypertensive heart disease, especially congestive heart failure, is as good as the prognosis for well-treated hypertensive patients who have never had this complication.

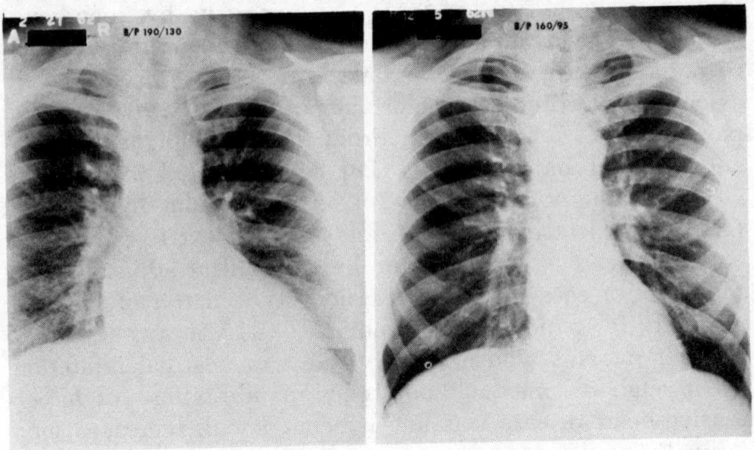

FIG. 6-1. Roentgenogram of chest of a 52-year-old man with severe hypertension and hypertensive heart disease. (*Left*) Before antihypertensive therapy was started (2/27/62). (*Right*) After control of hypertension (12/5/62). Note regression of cardiomegaly.

Management of Complicated Hypertension

Frequently, it is desirable to make modifications in usual treatment regimens and to observe special precautions in the use of certain drugs when hypertension is complicated. However, all "contraindications" are relative, and, in general, it is wiser to use drugs that are not in the "preferred" list in the tables when the preferred drugs are ineffective or cannot be tolerated than it is to permit uncontrolled hypertension to take its inexorable toll. Similarly, the dosage limits suggested in the tables may have to be exceeded on occasion to achieve the desired control of blood pressure.

Accelerated Hypertension

The presence of exudative retinopathy (exudates with or without hemorrhages) is so frequently associated with the rapid development of complications, especially renal failure, that hypertension in this situation is appropriately termed *accelerated hypertension.* When papilledema is also present, the prognosis is even worse, and, by definition, *malignant hypertension* exists.

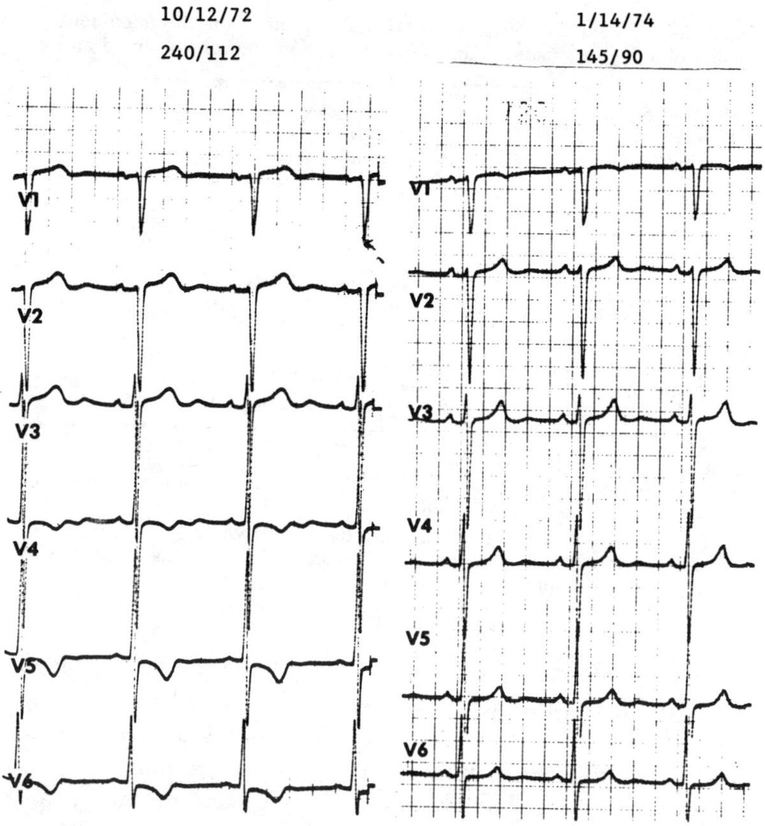

FIG. 6-2. Precordial leads of the electrocardiogram of a 63-year-old man with group 2 hypertension before (10/12/72) and during (1/14/74) effective antihypertensive treatment, showing reversion of ST–T abnormalities to normal. Note decrease in voltage of QRS.

Accelerated hypertension should be regarded as a medical emergency, requiring aggressive antihypertensive treatment, sometimes with parenteral agents initially to control hypertension rapidly until oral agents can be used effectively (Table 6-5). The rapidity with which blood pressure should be reduced is determined by the presence or absence of coexisting complications, which will be discussed subsequently. If no complications other than retinopathy are present, the goal should be to reduce blood pressure to normal range within 24–48 hours. The presence of left ventricular failure, hyperten-

Table 6-5. Parenteral and Oral Drug Regimen for Management of Accelerated Hypertension (Keith, Wagener, and Barker Groups 3 and 4)

Parenteral regimen[a]	
Reserpine	1–2 mg IM prn
Methyldopate	300–500 mg IV prn
Diazoxide	300 mg by IV push (within 15 seconds)
Oral	
Regimen 1[b]	
Diuretic[c]	
Propranolol	40 mg qid → 120 mg qid
Hydralazine	25 mg qid → 75 mg qid
Regimen 2[b]	
Diuretic[c]	
Methyldopa	250 mg qid → 500 mg qid
Guanethidine	25 mg qd → 100 mg qd

[a] Not always necessary (see test).
[b] Initiate therapy with all three drugs simultaneously and concomitantly with first dose of a parenteral agent if one is used.
[c] In the absence of renal failure, a thiazide derivative (e.g., chlorothiazide 500 mg bid or equivalent doses of a congener) or chlorthalidone (50 or 100 mg qd) is recommended.

sive encephalopathy, and (in some cases) intracerebral bleeding demands prompt reduction of blood pressure within minutes. On the other hand, if the patient also has acute cerebral or myocardial infarction or severe renal failure, it may be judicious to reduce blood pressure more gradually and perhaps to levels that are not absolutely normal.

Propranolol administered orally has been particularly useful in the control of accelerated hypertension, especially when used in conjunction with an oral diuretic and hydralazine (Table 6-5). It is by no means certain that the antihypertensive effect of propranolol is due to suppression of plasma renin activity, as postulated by Bühler et al [33]. In fact, many patients with accelerated hypertension do not have elevated plasma renin activity. Furthermore, if plasma renin activity is elevated, it usually decreases when blood pressure is reduced, irrespective of what drug or drugs are used. Thus, depression of plasma renin activity may be a nonspecific effect of blood pressure reduction in patients with accelerated hypertension.

Renal Failure

For a long time, physicians have been overly timid in their therapeutic approach to hypertension when chronic renal failure is present for fear that reduction of blood pressure will further compromise renal blood flow and thus cause more rapid deterioration of renal function. This cautious approach can no longer be justified, because uncontrolled hypertension begets more renal damage, which then makes hypertension worse. This vicious cycle can often be broken by appropriate antihypertensive therapy, with the result that azotemic patients whose hypertension is controlled may survive longer without the need for dialysis than if their hypertension had not been controlled [34, 35]. This is especially true if the serum creatinine is less than 8 mg per 100 ml when therapy is started.

It is not unusual for the blood urea nitrogen (BUN) and serum creatinine to increase when blood pressure is first reduced. However, this initial worsening of azotemia is often followed by improvement of renal function, manifested by a decrease in the concentration of BUN and serum creatinine, often to below the pretreatment levels [35].

Even when renal failure seems to be made worse, as evidenced by persistent increases in concentrations of BUN and serum creatinine, the physician should persist in his efforts to control hypertension, although it may be advisable to settle for blood pressure levels in the range of 150–160/90–100 mm Hg rather than absolute normotension. Sometimes, when azotemia is severe (e.g., BUN > 100 mg per 100 ml, or serum creatinine > 8 mg per 100 ml, or both), control of hypertension may seem to precipitate the need for dialysis. When this occurs, the physician should reassure the unfortunate patient and his family that the need for dialysis was imminent and inevitable anyhow, and, by keeping his blood pressure controlled, he has been protected from other ravages of hypertension that are more catastrophic and not so easily treated as renal failure, namely, dissecting aneurysm, cerebral hemorrhage, and cerebral or myocardial infarction.

Now that we have satisfactory dialysis techniques readily available to replace renal function, the physician is justified in being more concerned about other target organs of hypertension whose function cannot be replaced.

As a matter of fact, it is now well-accepted practice to remove both kidneys to control resistant and severe hypertension when all other measures have failed. In these cases, patients must remain on dialysis or receive a kidney transplant. Needless to say, this drastic measure should not be advised unless hypertension is severe, the kidneys are chronically and irreversibly diseased, and renal function is significantly impaired (creatinine clearance < 20 ml per minute). The peripheral plasma renin activity definitely should be elevated if bilateral nephrectomy is to be done, since it does not relieve hypertension for patients with normal or only slightly elevated plasma renin activity [36, 37].

Bilateral nephrectomy usually converts a severe, resistant, renin-dependent hypertension to a milder, volume-dependent, renoprival hypertension that can be managed successfully by appropriate fluid and sodium restriction and expert dialysis to avoid volume expansion. Sometimes, antihypertensive drugs are also needed, but usually small doses of propranolol or methyldopa with or without hydralazine are sufficient.

In the management of hypertension complicated by renal failure, care should be exercised in the choice of depressor drugs so that renal plasma flow will be jeopardized as little as possible when blood pressure is reduced (Table 6-6).

Of all the diuretics available, only furosemide and ethacrynic acid are effective when renal function is severely compromised (e.g., creatinine clearance < 20 ml per minute). In order to accomplish satisfactory diuresis in this situation, it usually is necessary to prescribe large doses of furosemide or ethacrynic acid, in the range of 350–1,500 mg daily. Gastrointestinal side effects occur so frequently when ethacrynic acid is administered to azotemic patients that furosemide is preferred. An additional benefit for the azotemic patient is that, unlike thiazide diuretics, neither furosemide nor ethacrynic acid directly reduces glomerular filtration rate.

Because of the danger of hyperkalemia, the distal tubular diuretics (spironolactone and triamterene) should be used with extreme caution, if at all, in azotemic patients. Hyperkalemia is a much greater threat to the azotemic patient than is hypokalemia.

Methyldopa, hydralazine, and diazoxide are particularly

Table 6-6. Modalities for Treatment of Hypertension Associated with Chronic Renal Failure

Diet
 Sodium and fluid restriction individualized to prevent expansion of plasma and extracellular fluid volume
Dialysis
 Ultrafiltration when necessary to correct volume expansion
Drugs—P. O.
 Mild or moderate hypertension (diastolic blood pressure 100–120 mm Hg)
  Furosemide[a] 160–1500 mg daily alone or in combination with
  Methyldopa 250 mg bid → 500 mg qid
   or
  Propranolol 40 mg tid → 80 mg qid
   Later add to regimen if necessary:
  Hydralazine 25 mg bid → 75 mg qid
 Severe hypertension (diastolic > 120 mm Hg)[b]
  Furosemide[a] 160–1,500 mg daily
   plus either:
  Methyldopa (250 mg qid → 500 mg qid) + hydralazine (25 mg qid → 75 mg qid)
   or
  Propranolol (40 mg → 120 mg qid) + hydralazine
  Add guanethidine 10 → 100 mg qd if necessary
Bilateral nephrectomy (see text)

[a] The dose of furosemide must be highly individualized; the more severe the hypertension and especially the more severe the renal failure, the greater the dose requirements. Total dose may be divided and administered two to four times daily. Furosemide should be withdrawn if severe oliguria or anuria persists. It is useless to incorporate furosemide in antihypertensive regimens for anephric patients.

[b] When hypertension is severe and intractable, initial treatment may include Furosemide, 80–120 mg IV, plus Diazoxide, 300 mg by IV push. This can be repeated as often as necessary to control blood pressure until oral regimens become effective.

useful in managing hypertension associated with renal failure, because they tend to maintain renal plasma flow at a higher level for any given decrement of blood pressure than do guanethidine or ganglion-blocking agents. The glomerular filtration rate may not be spared so much as renal plasma flow, because the filtration fraction usually decreases when methyldopa, hydralazine, or diazoxide is given to azotemic patients. Little is known about the effect of propranolol on renal function in azotemic hypertensive patients, but it does suppress renin activity, which may be important in managing hypertension associated with high renin levels. As stated previously, it is questionable whether propranolol's antihypertensive effect is related to its anti-renin effect. But in any event, clinical experience has shown that it is effective in controlling hypertension in azotemic patients, especially when used in conjunction with furosemide and hydralazine (Table 6-6).

Minoxidil is an investigational antihypertensive drug that acts like hydralazine to dilate resistance vessels directly. It is more potent than hydralazine and has been effective in controlling severe hypertension in end-stage renal failure for patients who otherwise would have required bilateral nephrectomy [38]. Like hydralazine, it should be used with propranolol and furosemide.

Cerebrovascular Disease

Hypertensive patients with clinical manifestations of cerebrovascular disease usually tolerate judicious antihypertensive therapy well despite evidence that cerebral autoregulation is not so effective in maintaining cerebral blood flow at lower levels of blood pressure in hypertensive patients as it is in normotensive persons [39]. The spectrum of cerebrovascular disease associated with hypertension is so wide and the indications for urgent treatment are so variable that each syndrome will be considered separately.

HYPERTENSIVE ENCEPHALOPATHY. Hypertensive encephalopathy is a medical emergency demanding prompt reduction of blood pressure to normal levels. Diazoxide or sodium nitroprusside is the drug of choice (Table 6-7). Usually, it is advisable to administer furosemide, 80 mg IV, with each dose of diazoxide to prevent fluid retention. The blood pressure should be maintained at normal levels with parenteral agents until an effective oral regimen can be established.

Reserpine and methyldopa are not recommended for parenteral use in treating this acute crisis, because they have a slow onset of action (2–3 hours), and they produce enough drowsiness and somnolence to interfere with the clinical evaluation of the patient's level of consciousness.

Table 6-7. Regimens for Management of Acute Hypertensive Encephalopathy

Give:
Furosemide 80 mg IV (repeat at least q12h)
plus one of the following:
Diazoxide 300 mg by IV push prn to keep blood pressure < 170/110
or
Sodium nitroprusside 100 mg/L by continuous IV infusion
or
Trimethaphan camsylate 1,000 mg/L by continuous IV infusion
or
Pentolinium 1–5 mg IM prn
or
Hydralazine 10–20 mg IM prn
Avoid if possible (see text):
Reserpine
Methyldopa

INTRACEREBRAL HEMORRHAGE. There is wide divergence of opinion about the advisability of acutely reducing blood pressure for patients with hypertensive cerebral hemorrhage (intracerebral hematoma). Some physicians, usually neurosurgeons, advocate reducing blood pressure promptly and maintaining it at low normotensive or sometimes even hypotensive levels. For this purpose, sodium nitroprusside is the agent of choice (Table 6-8). Other physicians, usually neurologists, take the position that the hypertension is compensatory, to maintain cerebral blood flow to areas of the brain surrounding the hematoma, where intense vasospasm is often demonstrated by angiography. No well-controlled studies have been carried out to resolve this dilemma.

It has been a clinical impression that patients with intracerebral bleeding whose hypertension is controlled do better than those who do not receive antihypertensive therapy. Admittedly, the prognosis is poor, with or without treatment.

An infusion of sodium nitroprusside is used to reduce blood pressure to or toward normal gradually over a period of 10–30 minutes, and if this reduction is not accompanied by deterioration of the patient's neurologic status, it should be maintained. On the other hand, if the neurologic deficit seems to worsen as blood pressure is reduced, the infusion can be stopped or

Table 6-8. Regimens for Management of Acute Cerebral Hemorrhage (Intracerebral Hematoma)

Give:
- Furosemide 80 mg IV (repeat at least q12h)
  - *plus one of the following:*
- Sodium nitroprusside 100 mg/L by IV infusion[a]
  - *or*
- Trimethaphan camsylate 1,000 mg/L by IV infusion[a]
  - *or*
- Hydralazine 10–20 mg IM prn
  - *or*
- Pentolinium 1–5 mg IM prn

Avoid if possible (see text):
- Reserpine
- Methyldopa
- Diazoxide

[a] The blood pressure should be reduced gradually over a 30-minute period by precise adjustment of the rate of infusion. The goal should be normotension unless the neurologic deficit worsens, in which case the rate of infusion can be slowed or stopped, allowing the blood pressure to rise.

appropriately slowed, and the blood pressure will rise almost immediately (Table 6-8).

Diazoxide is not recommended in this situation because it has to be given by IV push, following which the blood pressure drops precipitously and may stay at normotensive levels for 6–12 hours after the injection. This would require administration of a pressor agent if the patient seemed to get worse when the blood pressure fell. Some investigators advocate administering smaller doses of diazoxide (e.g., 100 mg) by IV push every 5 minutes until the blood pressure is at the desired level. In this manner the blood pressure is reduced more gradually, which is desirable in treating hypertension associated with acute intracranial bleeding.

For reasons already mentioned in the preceding section, reserpine and methyldopa are not recommended for parenteral administration in patients with acute cerebral hemorrhage.

CEREBRAL INFARCTION. During the acute phase of cerebral infarction ("stroke in evolution"), and for the first two or three weeks after a completed stroke, it is best not to administer antihypertensive agents unless the blood pressure is greater than 180 mm Hg systolic, or 110 mm Hg diastolic, or both. If blood pressure exceeds these levels, antihypertensive therapy should be administered orally. Some recommended regimens are listed in Table 6-9. The goal of therapy is to keep the blood pressure in the range of 150–180 mm Hg systolic and 95–110 mm Hg diastolic until the clinical situation has stabilized. Orthostatic hypotension should be avoided if at all possible, and for this reason, ganglion-blocking agents and guanethidine are not recommended unless blood pressure cannot be controlled without them.

If the patient is unconscious or cannot swallow, antihypertensive agents will have to be given parenterally for a while. For this purpose, hydralazine or pentolinium may be given intramuscularly or methyldopate given intravenously, provided the latter's sedative properties do not obscure the neurologic evaluation of the patient. Furosemide should be given intravenously in doses of 40–80 mg at least twice daily to prevent fluid retention. When given by itself, hydralazine sometimes causes a reflex tachycardia and increases cardiac output, which can be detrimental if the patient has preexisting heart disease. Under these circumstances, methyldopate or propranolol can be administered intravenously, or pentolinium can be administered intramuscularly to block the reflex effect of hydralazine on the heart. If pentolinium is employed, it is important to keep the patient recumbent, without elevation of the head of the bed, to avoid orthostatic hypotension.

During the acute phase of a cerebral infarction, especially in the brain stem, hypertension may occasionally be severe (> 240/140 mm Hg). When this occurs, sodium nitroprusside should be administered in sufficient dosage to decrease blood pressure gradually (within 20–30 minutes) to levels approximating 180/110 mm Hg. This requires expert titration of the infusion rate. As an alternative, small doses of hydralazine or pentolinium may be given intramuscularly, or trimethaphan may be given as a continuous infusion. Like pentolinium, trimethaphan is a ganglion-blocking agent and may produce profound orthostatic hypotension; thus, the precautions described in the previous paragraph must be taken to avoid this in patients who have had acute cerebrovascular accidents.

Once a patient has recovered from the acute phase of cere-

Table 6-9. Management of Hypertension Associated with Acute Cerebral Infarction

Diastolic < 110 mm Hg

No treatment for 3 weeks

Diastolic 110–125 mm Hg

orally

Diuretic[a] with or without { Propranolol 40 mg bid → 120 mg qid *or* Methyldopa 250 mg bid → 500 mg qid } + Hydralazine 25 mg bid → 75 mg qid

Diastolic > 125 mm Hg

Diuretic[a] + propranolol + hydralazine

Diuretic[a] + methyldopa + guanethidine[b] (10 mg qd → 50 mg qd)

[a] A thiazide derivative (chlorothiazide 500 mg bid, hydroclorothiazide 50 mg bid) or chlorthalidone 50 mg qd.

[b] Use cautiously to avoid orthostatic hypotension (see text).

bral infarction and the neurologic deficit has stabilized (usually three weeks after the acute event), hypertension should be treated with the same regimens that would be used for hypertensive patients who have never had a stroke (Table 6-10). The goal should be to normalize the blood pressure (< 140/90 mm Hg). Ideally, drugs that cause orthostatic hypotension, such as guanethidine and ganglion-blocking agents, should be avoided, and usually this is possible. However, most patients with old cerebral infarcts tolerate orthostatic hypotension surprisingly well. If it becomes necessary to use orthostatic agents to control blood pressure, patients should be warned about rising from the seated or recumbent position too rapidly. Guanethidine was an important ingredient in the regimens used by Marshall [19] for his patients with hypertension and completed strokes. He demonstrated that the treated patients lived longer and had fewer recurrences of stroke than did the untreated patients.

The *lacunar state*, characterized by gait disturbances, bilateral neurologic signs, and pseudobulbar palsy (the syndrome of "little strokes"), seems to be peculiarly related to hypertension and is due to multiple tiny infarcts (lacunae) in the white matter of the hemispheres, brain stem, and cerebellum. These patients seem to tolerate reduction of blood pressure less well than do patients who have had a discrete cerebral infarction. Yet control of blood pressure is the only hope for arresting the progress of this syndrome. The goal should

Table 6-10. Management of Hypertension Associated with Remote Cerebral Infarction or Hypertensive or Ischemic Heart Disease or Both

Diastolic 90–120 mm Hg	*orally*
Diuretic[a] with or without	Methyldopa 250 mg bid → 500 mg qid *or* Propranolol 40 mg bid → 120 mg qid
Later add third agent:	Hydralazine 25 mg bid → 75 mg qid
Diastolic > 120 mm Hg	
Diuretic[a] + propranolol + hydralazine *or* Diuretic[a] + methyldopa Add guanethidine (10 mg → 100 mg qd) if necessary	

[a] A thiazide derivative (e.g., chlorothiazide 500 mg bid or hydrochlorothiazide 50 mg bid) or chlorthalidone 50 mg qd.

be to keep the blood pressure as nearly normal as the patient can tolerate, using the same regimens as suggested for patients with completed strokes (Table 6-10).

TRANSIENT ISCHEMIC ATTACKS. Transient ischemic attacks (TIA) often improve when hypertension is controlled. The conventional antihypertensive regimens recommended for patients with completed strokes should be employed (Table 6-10). If possible, orthostatic hypotension should be avoided by instituting the measures described in the preceding section. The concern that reduction of blood pressure for patients with TIA might precipitate a stroke has not been substantiated by clinical experience. On the other hand, control of hypertension has not been shown to prevent cerebral infarction, which ultimately occurs in 15–30 percent of patients with TIA. Consequently, treatment, either medical (anticoagulants or aspirin) or surgical, directed at the atherosclerotic lesion itself, is also sometimes indicated.

Cardiac Complications

Because of difficulties in therapeutic approach, it is convenient to divide the cardiac complications of hypertension into those due to hypertensive heart disease and those due to atherosclerotic coronary artery disease. In actual practice, however, the two often coexist, making therapeutic decisions more difficult.

HYPERTENSIVE HEART DISEASE. Acute left ventricular failure from hypertensive heart disease is one of the most gratifying medical emergencies to treat, because a salutary response to rapid reduction of blood pressure is usually obtained. Blood pressure should be reduced to normal by using parenteral agents, including furosemide, intravenously. Diazoxide, sodium nitroprusside, or trimethaphan is the agent of choice. Because diazoxide is more convenient to give and requires less monitoring than do infusions of sodium nitroprusside or trimethaphan, it is usually chosen (Table 6-11).

Prompt reduction of blood pressure enormously decreases the work load of the failing left ventricle and is vastly more important than administering a digitalis glycoside parenterally.

Table 6-11. Emergency Management of Hypertension Associated with Acute Left Ventricular Failure

1. Diuretic:
   a. Furosemide (Lasix) 40–80 mg IV
      or
   b. Ethacrynic acid (Edecrin) 50–100 mg IV
2. Antihypertensive:
   a. Diazoxide (Hyperstat) 300 mg IV (within 15 seconds)
      or
   b. Sodium nitroprusside (Nipride) 100 mg per liter IV
      or
   c. Trimethaphan (Arfonad) 1,000 mg per liter IV
      or
   d. Pentolinium (Ansolysen) 1–2 mg IM
3. Lanatoside C (Cedilanid IV) (not always necessary)
4. Oxygen, morphine, rotating tourniquets, venesection (phlebotomy)
5. Sodium restriction

In fact, most of the time it is possible to restore cardiac compensation without using digitalis at all. If it is given during the acute episode of left ventricular failure, it can be stopped once the blood pressure has been controlled. Parenteral antihypertensive agents can be discontinued as soon as an effective oral regimen has been established (Table 6-10). (See Chapter 5.)

If congestive heart failure is not fulminating, therapy may be initiated with oral agents unless the blood pressure is extremely high (> 200/130 mm Hg), in which case it is usually prudent to use parenteral agents initially.

While cardiac decompensation is a well-known contraindication to the use of propranolol, this drug can be included in oral regimens if the heart failure is due only to hypertensive heart disease and if the blood pressure is effectively reduced by the regimen. In this situation, reduction of left ventricular work load by decreasing blood pressure outweighs the depressing effects of propranolol on the myocardium. Furthermore, the concomitant administration of digitalis is recommended when propranolol is to be used for treating patients with hypertensive heart disease and left ventricular failure, at least until blood pressure is normalized and cardiac compensation is restored, because digitalis protects the myocardium against the negative inotropic effect of propranolol.

Moderate dietary sodium restriction (2 gm daily) is advisable for patients with hypertensive heart disease who have or have had congestive heart failure. An oral diuretic must be included in every antihypertensive regimen. This is especially true for patients with hypertensive heart disease with or without congestive heart failure.

Conventional antihypertensive regimens are recommended for patients who have manifestations of hypertensive heart disease (cardiac enlargement, atrial abnormalities, the changes of left ventricular hypertrophy on ECG, or a fourth heart sound) without overt failure. There should be no hesitancy about including propranolol in the regimens for such patients, provided blood pressure is effectively controlled (Table 6-10).

Hydralazine may be prescribed for patients with hypertensive heart disease if a sympathetic depressant agent (such as reserpine, methyldopa, guanethidine, or propranolol) is included in the same regimen to block the reflex tachycardia and increase in cardiac output that often occur if hydralazine is used by itself.

ATHEROSCLEROTIC HEART DISEASE. Mild to moderate hypertension (140–180 mm Hg systolic, or 90–110 mm Hg diastolic, or both) probably should not be treated during episodes of impending myocardial infarction or immediately after an acute myocardial infarction unless congestive heart failure is also present, in which case judicious use of sodium nitroprusside is preferred because it greatly reduces the afterload on the ventricle [40]. Hypotension should be avoided.

Acute coronary insufficiency with or without actual infarction is sometimes accompanied by severe hypertension (> 240 mm Hg systolic, or 140 mm Hg diastolic, or both) that seems to be caused, perhaps reflexly, by myocardial ischemia [41]. Needless to say, such a burden on an ischemic left ventricle is unnecessary and dangerous. This hypertensive crisis should be treated with reserpine intramuscularly, methyldopa intravenously, or sodium nitroprusside by intravenous infusion. Drastic reduction of blood pressure to normal levels in this situation seems unwarranted. The goal should be to keep the blood pressure in a moderate range (150–180 mm Hg systolic and 95–110 mm Hg diastolic). Reserpine and methyldopa reduce blood pressure gradually over a period of 2–3 hours, and the accompanying sedation is beneficial for the apprehensive patient with acute myocardial ischemia. With expert titration of a sodium nitroprusside infusion, the blood pressure can also be gently reduced and maintained at the desired level.

An oral antihypertensive regimen (Table 6-10) should be prescribed for patients with impending infarction or after acute myocardial infarction when blood pressure exceeds 180/110 mm Hg. If more prompt reduction of blood pressure seems desirable, the parenteral regimens described in the previous paragraph are recommended.

After the infarction is more than three or four weeks old, hypertension of any magnitude should be treated, and the goal of therapy should be normotension ($< 140/90$ mm Hg). Standard regimens should be used (Table 6-10). (See also Chapter 5.) Hydralazine should not be used alone for patients with atherosclerotic heart disease for the same reason that it is not recommended for patients with congestive heart failure (see p. 171). Inclusion of propranolol in the regimen is especially indicated when angina pectoris is present, because propranolol is both an antihypertensive and antianginal drug.

There is naturally some concern that reducing blood pressure in patients who also have atherosclerotic occlusive disease of the coronary arteries may actually decrease coronary blood flow as the head of the pressure in the aorta declines. Frequently forgotten is the fact that reduction of arterial blood pressure also decreases the work load, and consequently the oxygen requirement, of the left ventricle. If coronary perfusion is decreased more than oxygen requirements, then antihypertensive treatment will have an unfavorable effect. Fortunately, the reverse is almost always true, namely, that oxygen requirements are reduced more than coronary flow. Undoubtedly, this explains why angina is usually less frequent when hypertension is controlled than when it is not.

Conclusions

The presence of any cardiovascular or renal complications or both compromises prognosis for the hypertensive patient. Consequently, antihypertensive therapy should be initiated before complications occur. However, the presence of complications should not be a deterrent to treatment, because effective control of blood pressure improves the outlook for the hypertensive patient with complications, although the prognosis is not as good as if complications had never occurred.

References

1. Freis, E., et al. Veterans Administration Cooperative Study Group on Antihypertensive Agents: Effects of treatment on morbidity in hypertension. I. Results in patients with diastolic blood pressures averaging 115 through 129 mm Hg. *J. A. M. A.* 202:1028, 1967.
2. Freis, E., et al. Veterans Administration Cooperative Study Group on Antihypertensive Agents: Effects of treatment on morbidity in hypertension. II. Results in patients with diastolic blood pressures averaging 90 through 114 mm Hg. *J. A. M. A.* 213:1143, 1970.
3. Veterans Administration Cooperative Study Group on Antihypertensive Agents. Effects of treatment on morbidity in hypertension. III. Influence of age, diastolic pressure, and prior cardiovascular disease; further analysis of side effects. *Circulation* 45:991, 1972.
4. Smirk, F. H. Observations on the mortality of 270 treated and 199 untreated retinal grade I and II hypertensive patients followed in all instances for five years. *N. Z. Med. J.* 63:413, 1964.
5. Mathisen, H. S., Löken, H., Brox, D., and Stenbaek, O. The prognosis in long term and treated and "untreated" essential hypertension. *Acta Med. Scand.* 185:253, 1969.
6. Breslin, D. J., Gifford, R. W., Jr., and Fairbairn, J. F., II. Essential hypertension: A twenty-year follow-up study. *Circulation* 33:87, 1966.
7. Simpson, F. O., and Gilchrist, A. R. Prognosis in untreated hypertensive vascular disease. *Scott. Med. J.* 3:1, 1958.
8. Keith, N. M., Wagener, H. P., and Barker, N. W. Some different types of essential hypertension: Their course and prognosis. *Am. J. Med. Sci.* 197:332, 1939.
9. Kincaid-Smith, P., McMichael, J., and Murphy, E. A. The clinical course and pathology of hypertension with papilloedema (malignant hypertension). *Q. J. Med.* 27:117, 1958.
10. Harrington, M., Kincaid-Smith, P., and McMichael, J. Results of Treatment in Malignant Hypertension. *Br. Med. J.* 1:969, 1959.
11. Dustan, H. P., et al. The effectiveness of long-term treatment of malignant hypertension. *Circulation* 18:644, 1958.

12. Breckenridge, A., Dollery, C. T., and Parry, E. H. O. Prognosis of treated hypertension. *Q. J. Med.* 39:411, 1970.
13. Mohler, E. R., Jr., and Freis, E. D. Five-year survival of patients with malignant hypertension treated with antihypertensive agents. *Am. Heart J.* 60:329, 1960.
14. North, J. D. K., Williams, J. C. P., and Howie, R. N. Severe Hypertension treated with ganglion-blocking drugs in a general hospital. *Br. Med. J.* 1:1426, 1961.
15. Farmer, R. G., Gifford, R. W., Jr., and Hines, E. A., Jr. Effect of Medical Treatment of Severe Hypertension. *Arch. Intern. Med.* 112:118, 1963.
16. Perry, M. Survival of treated hypertensive patients. Therapeutic grand rounds No. 20. *J. A. M. A.* 210:890, 1969.
17. Millikan, C. H. The stroke-prone profile. Current concepts of cerebrovascular disease. *Stroke* 4:17, 1969.
18. Hypertension-Stroke Cooperative Study Group. Effect of antihypertensive treatment on stroke recurrence. *J. A. M. A.* 229: 409, 1974.
19. Marshall, J. A trial of long-term hypotensive therapy in cerebrovascular disease. *Lancet* 1:10, 1964.
20. Carter, A. B. Hypotensive therapy in stroke survivors. *Lancet* 1:487, 1970.
21. Beevers, D. G., et al. Antihypertensive treatment and the course of established cerebral vascular disease. *Lancet* 1:1407, 1973.
22. Hamilton, M. The need for early reduction of blood pressure: Illustrated by the long-term results of treatment of hypertension. *N. Z. Med. J.* 67:275, 1968.
23. Sokolow, M., and Perloff, D. The prognosis of essential hypertension treated conservatively. *Circulation* 23:697, 1961.
24. Frank, C. W., et al. Prognosis of men with coronary heart disease as related to blood pressure. *Circulation* 38:432, 1968.
25. Leishman, A. W. D. Hypertension—Treated and untreated; a study of 400 cases. *Br. Med. J.* 1:1361, 1959.
26. Moyer, J. H., and Heider, C. Some observations on morbidity and prognosis as affected by antihypertensive therapy in patients with essential hypertension. *Am. J. Cardiol.* 9:920, 1962.
27. Oxman, H. A., et al. The effect of treatment of hypertension on prognosis in patients with clinical ischemic heart disease (Abst.). *Circulation* (Suppl. II) 45 and 46:104, 1972.
28. Hodge, J. V., and Smirk, F. H. The effect of drug treatment of hypertension on distribution of deaths from various causes. *Am. Heart J.* 73:441, 1967.
29. Kannel, W. B., et al. Electrocardiographic left ventricular hypertrophy and risk of coronary heart disease. *Ann. Intern. Med.* 72:813, 1970.
30. Kannel, W. B., et al. Role of blood pressure in the develop-

ment of congestive heart failure. *N. Engl. J. Med.* 287:782, 1972.

31. Dern, P. L., et al. Serial electrocardiographic changes in treated hypertensive patients with reference to voltage criteria, mean QRS vectors, and QRS–T angle. *Circulation* 36:823, 1967.
32. Poblett, P. F., et al. Effect of treatment on morbidity in hypertension (Veterans Administration Cooperative Study on Antihypertensive Agents). *Circulation* 48:481, 1973.
33. Bühler, F. R., et al. Propranolol inhibition of renin secretion; a specific approach to diagnosis and treatment of renin-dependent hypertensive diseases. *N. Engl. J. Med.* 287:1209, 1972.
34. Woods, J. W., Blythe, W. B., and Huffines, W. D. Management of malignant hypertension complicated by renal insufficiency. A follow-up study. *N. Engl. J. Med.* 241:10, 1974.
35. Mroczek, W. J., et al. The value of aggressive therapy in the hypertensive patient with azotemia. *Circulation* 40:893, 1969.
36. Vertes, V., et al. Hypertension in end-stage renal disease. *N. Engl. J. Med.* 280:978, 1969.
37. Weidmann, P., et al. Plasma renin activity and blood pressure in terminal renal failure. *N. Engl. J. Med.* 285:757, 1971.
38. Pettinger, W. A., and Mitchell, H. C. Minoxidil–An alternative to nephrectomy for refractory hypertension. *N. Engl. J. Med.* 289:167, 1973.
39. Strandgaard, S., et al. Autoregulation of brain circulation in severe arterial hypertension. *Br. Med. J.* 1:507, 1973.
40. Franciosa, J. A., et al. Improved left ventricular function during nitroprusside infusion in acute myocardial infarction. *Lancet* 1:650, 1972.
41. Horwitz, D., and Sjoerdsma, A. Some Inter-relationships Between Elevation of Blood Pressure and Angina Pectoris. *Proceedings of the Council for High Blood Pressure Research of the American Heart Association,* Vol. 13, 1965. P. 39.

7. Patient Management Problems: Questions and Answers

Ray W. Gifford, Jr., J. Caulie Gunnells, Jr., Arthur H. Hayes, William L. McGuffin, Jr., Marvin Moser, and Louis Tobian

The following series of questions and answers from the Tarrytown Conference may help to clarify some practical management problems encountered in clinical practice.

QUESTION: Dr. Moser, what should I tell my hypertensive patients about diet, exercise, use of alcohol, or cigarettes? How much should they change their life-style?

DR. MOSER:

1. Once the patient's blood pressure is controlled, he should be able to participate in any kind of sports activity, such as jogging, tennis, and so forth.
2. With regard to cigarettes: There is no evidence that moderate use of cigarettes affects blood pressure, but chain smoking does increase blood pressure through a catecholamine release. If you are concerned about other risk factors, then cigarette smoking should be prohibited, since it is a major independent risk factor in cardiovascular disease.
3. Alcohol in moderation never hurt anyone.
4. There is no question that lowering sodium intake to a great degree (under 500 mg a day) will lower blood pressure, but most patients will not stay on a diet very low in sodium. A low-carbohydrate diet plus a low-sodium diet would be even more effective, but patient compliance to such a program is also poor. Most patients can be managed without a loss of diuretic effect by merely restricting their intake be-

low the average United States intake of about 10 gm to an average of 5 or 6 gm a day. Dr. Tobian apparently finds this approach acceptable.

QUESTION: Dr. Gifford, you mentioned furosemide quite a bit in the management of hypertensive encephalopathy and in the management of renal failure with hypertension. Would you comment about furosemide in the usual case of hypertension. Is it any better than a thiazide?

DR. GIFFORD: No, I don't think it is. As a matter of fact, it presents some of the same problems that spironolactone does. It takes a bigger dose, more tablets a day, and therefore is more expensive. In several control studies that have been done and in another still in progress, 80 mg of furosemide twice a day was not equal to 50 mg of hydrochlorothiazide twice a day in its antihypertensive potency.

The key point here may be the short duration of action of furosemide. In the unfinished study I mentioned, the dose of furosemide has been increased to 40 mg four times a day, comparing it to 50 mg of hydrochlorothiazide twice a day. I'll guess that they will have equal potency, but this is four tablets versus two. You have to spread them out through the day because furosemide has a very short duration of action, and I really think that it has no advantage and some disadvantage in the management of the *average* patient with hypertension.

In those patients who remain resistant in spite of the thiazide, you can occasionally get a good result by giving increasing doses of furosemide—up to 240–300 mg a day—for a short period of time, to bring the plasma volume back down; but this is a different situation.

DR. MOSER: There are other cases that won't respond when a full dose of a thiazide is given, and it is useful to add furosemide, 40–80 mg every second or third day, to gain a good response.

QUESTION: A question about the dosage of guanethidine.

DR. GIFFORD: The dosage can be anywhere from 12.5 mg a day to as high as 350 mg a day. The dosage should be increased until the blood pressure is lowered. Either you get side effects or you get the blood pressure down to where you want it. That is a rule that we should follow completely in all antihypertensive therapy.

QUESTION: What about the use of antihypertensive drugs in the pregnant woman or in the woman of childbearing age? Are there any data on genetic effects of long-term diuretic therapy, or any dilatory side effects?

DR. HAYES: There is not much evidence of any adverse genetic effects of the thiazides. The classification of hypertension in pregnancy (of eclampsia, or preeclampsia with or without preexisting or superimposed hypertension) attempts to set some guidelines for therapy, but treatment is terribly difficult. I think that there are some general rules.

The patient who is hypertensive before pregnancy clearly will have a greater fetal salvage and a decrease in maternal mortality if the blood pressure is controlled during pregnancy; and here, very often, the therapy has to be directed towards non-drugs, such as bed rest, salt restriction, and so on. Diuretic therapy is very controversial, and there are some reports that thiazides are not helpful and may be injurious to the fetus if used chronically in hypertension. Some experts believe that salt restriction is much better.

The only drugs that I know of that would be strictly contraindicated in the pregnant woman with hypertension, even in a crisis, are the ganglionic-blocking agents, because they regularly produce meconium ileus and a high fetal loss. These are rarely used.

DR. GIFFORD: Thiazides are used so much in pregnant women, not just for hypertension but for edema, and so on. Thousands of pregnant women have received thiazides, and if there were genetic effects, it would certainly have been recognized. I think it is ridiculous to go around the mulberry bush again with the obstetricians. They treat in one way, and other doctors treat in another way.

DR. MOSER: It's true that we're right back to where we first started from in the 1930s and 1940s. Blood pressure elevations in the second or third trimester are being treated with bed rest and sedation without diuretics. Patients are put to bed and sedated. Long hospitalizations and the psychic trauma of taking the woman out of the house, and so on, seem unnecessary when diuretics have been quite successful. If drug therapy fails to lower pressure and reduce edema and albuminuria, bed rest and sedation can always be used. It seems to me that our experience in the early 1950s was very good when diuretics were used.

DR. TOBIAN: Wait a minute. Bed rest for reasons that aren't clear has an extremely beneficial influence in preeclampsia. If you've ever had experience with preeclampsia, you have to admit that. I remember doing a project on preeclampsia, and if I didn't start the study within a day of the patient's coming into the hospital, the preeclampsia would disappear. I don't think there is any question that bed rest has a terrific effect. Today, a lot of women are being put to bed for two, four, six, and eight weeks and being treated that way instead of having their pressure handled in other ways. Bed rest obviously works.

DR. MOSER: Obviously a problem that may have several solutions. Dr. Tobian, do you use diuretics in addition to bed rest?

DR. TOBIAN: In the presence of edema I probably would. I don't believe that we can ignore your and Dr. Gifford's experiences with toxemia of pregnancy either. We probably should remain cautious and await further data about diuretics and pregnancy.

QUESTION: Dr. Gunnells, would you comment on blood pressure and the pill?

DR. GUNNELLS: This is certainly a low-incidence problem, but it is one that you have to deal with. I think that every young woman who comes into the office who has hypertension must be asked if she is on oral contraceptive medications. If so, before going into an expensive evaluation, I stop the medication and wait three months. You have to wait a minimum of three months before the affect of the pill is really dissipated. If she remains hypertensive, you go ahead from there. Just one quick point: There is nothing magic about the pill. If you are concerned about hypertension, remember that it may occur with estrogens when given as replacement therapy in older women. There have been reports of hypertensive encephalopathy in patients receiving estrogens.

QUESTION: Dr. Tobian, would you instruct a normotensive patient with a negative family history and no other risk factors in the use of table salt? What would you tell him? Do you think there is a risk of developing hypertension with a negative family history and no other risk factors if you are a heavy salt user?

DR. TOBIAN: I guess a person cannot be sure he doesn't have hypertension in his family unless he checks very carefully. In all honesty, you would have to tell him to go easy on salt because he couldn't be certain that there was no hypertension in his family.

DR. MOSER: There are studies, as you know, in different population groups that demonstrate that those with a high salt intake do have an increased level of blood pressure—not necessarily hypertensive blood pressure, but pressure in the high normal range. They might average 135/85–90 mm Hg where similar people with a lower salt intake might average 125/85 mm Hg. They might, therefore, not be detected and labeled as hypertensive. I would advise people to use salt in moderation and certainly not to ingest up to the 15–20 gm or more a day that some people do in Japan and the Bahamas.

DR. TOBIAN: If you compare blood volumes of people who take in 10 as opposed to 200 mEq of salt a day, the blood volumes will be quite different. I think one of the reasons people talk about 100 mEq or 5 gm is that the part of the population that doesn't eat any more than that per day practically have no hypertension, even in those who are susceptible. If you are not susceptible, it probably doesn't make any difference how much salt you eat.

There have been studies that show if you eat a huge amount of salt and are hypertensive, you can negate or reduce the effect of a reasonable dose of thiazides. The other point is that you probably get a little more hypokalemia on thiazides if you have a huge amount of salt. Over millions of years, human beings were struggling to get enough salt. For about 300 years they have been acquiring the opposite problem. From the evolutionary point of view, we weren't really designed to have large amounts of salt.

DR. MOSER: You have to take in over 18–20 gm a day of salt to break through the usual diuretic effects of the thiazides. If we could restrict people and have them follow a rigid regimen, they would certainly be better off on a very minimal sodium intake and a minimal carbohydrate intake, but we can't do it in most individuals, and these kinds of life-style restrictions are probably not necessary if drugs are used properly.

QUESTION: Why shouldn't an arteriogram rather than an IVP be the first screening test in a patient whom you suspect has renovascular disease. If you do an IVP in a patient under 20 and it is negative, you know that there are 15–20 percent false negatives, and you will do an arteriogram anyway. Why not skip the IVP?

DR. GIFFORD: I do that all the time. In my mind, if I say that this patient needs a renal angiogram, I don't give a darn what the IVP shows. I frequently do the angiogram and skip the patient's IVP.

DR. MOSER: But only in patients where some work-up is clearly indicated. I agree that in an 18-year-old with a diastolic of 110 mm Hg or higher and a bruit in the abdomen, you would never stop with an IVP. Ordinarily, of course, we like to do noninvasive procedures first.

QUESTION: If a woman is already hypertensive and under medical control, is there any reason why she shouldn't be on the pill? What is your experience with that?

DR. GUNNELLS: There are lots of patients on antihypertensive drugs who are taking the pill and are doing just fine. I just leave them alone.

DR. GIFFORD: I would, too. You have to watch them because you are really at fault if something happens and they develop malignant hypertension and you haven't seen them for six months. So you would watch them a little more closely than the usual patient. I have patients on the pill whose blood pressure is well controlled on antihypertensive agents.

QUESTION: Do you use propranolol in all these individuals because of its renin-lowering effect if you put them on the pill?

DR. GIFFORD: No, not necessarily, but I use propranolol a great deal anyhow.

QUESTION: Does anyone use acetazolamide for the treatment of hypertension?

DR. MOSER: Not in hypertension. It is a very mild diuretic agent. We have better drugs available. It is useful in glaucoma.

QUESTION: What treatment should be given to patients with occasionally elevated blood pressure, that is, with casually elevated blood pressures to about 160/90?

DR. MOSER: All of us would agree that these people are at increased risk for cardiovascular morbidity and mortality. They should be followed, and if they spike occasionally, they probably should be started on minimal diuretic therapy and/or rauwolfia or propranolol three to four times a week at first, with a gradual increase in therapy until blood pressure is reduced to normal even during times of anxiety or on casual determinations.

DR. TOBIAN: I would try to get them on a lower salt intake if I could persuade them to do it. If they continue to have spiking blood pressures, which most of them do, I often put them on a minute dose of a long-acting thiazide-type drug such as chlorthalidone.

QUESTION: In a patient with severe renal insufficiency with a creatinine clearance of 10 ml per minute, would you give furosemide in large doses, in divided doses, or in single doses? How often would you repeat diazoxide safely?

DR. GIFFORD: I usually divide the dose of furosemide into three to four doses a day; in other words, a total of 240–300 mg divided into three or four doses. In a few patients, there seems to be a better diuresis if you give them a bigger dose twice a day or maybe the whole dose once a day; but, in general, it is best to use this short-acting drug frequently.

Regarding diazoxide in these patients: Dr. Finnerty has shown that if you give large doses of furosemide, you can keep the pressure down with diazoxide. Every time the blood pressure gets above a certain level (160/90–170/110 mm Hg), start them with diazoxide again. We have been able to rescue quite a few of these patients with rather advanced renal failure, and we have had surprisingly long survivals. After 8–10 days, you switch them over to an oral regimen—methyldopa, reserpine, hydralazine, and/or guanethidine—and continue with a high dose of furosemide. We give enough furosemide to insure a urine output of a liter a day. This way, I think we have been able to have a remarkable record in these patients with rather advanced renal insufficiency.

There is just one comment I would like to make about diazoxide as compared with trimethaphan or nitroprusside. Diazoxide is so easy to use, comparatively speaking, in terms of monitoring, that we have found in the hospital, especially among house officers, that they can become lazy and just keep giving it. If you have to watch a patient and stay up all night and come running when the nurse calls because the nitroprusside has gotten the pressure too low and the trimethaphan is not right, you'll want to get the patient on oral medication as quickly as possible. This is a more correct approach.

We have had a couple of referred patients who have been on diazoxide for as long as 10 days around the clock and on nothing else. I think that you have to be careful that you don't use this drug indefinitely. It changes the parameters.

DR. MOSER: Diazoxide has certainly simplified management in hospitals that do not have an adequate house staff.

There are patients who develop tolerance after the second or third dose of diazoxide, but when it works, it works very well. If it doesn't work after the second or third dose, you switch to something else. Usually, after a large dose of furosemide (80–120 mg IV), sensitvity will be enhanced as plasma volume is reduced. Nitroprusside might produce good results, but its use requires constant monitoring.

QUESTION: Is there any indication for the use of isosorbid in hypertensive patients with angina? I would imagine you use isosorbide or any other antianginal drug just the way you do with normotensive patients.

DR. GIFFORD: I think that there is little evidence that any of those things are good. That's right! Lower the blood pressure first. Frequently, angina disappears.

QUESTION: What do you do in a family where lots of people have had hypertension and where you follow or have been referred a patient who has had a blood pressure elevation for 15 or 20 years. He seems to be perfectly fine and doing well, and he tells you that his mother and father are 84 and have had high blood pressure. Do you ignore him? Do you say he is lucky or do you treat him? He is 58 years old and his pressure is 180/120 mm Hg. He has some voltage criteria of LVH and no proteinuria.

DR. TOBIAN: I'd treat him.

QUESTION: When do you use allopurinol if the uric acid is increased?

DR. MOSER: Obviously, if someone is having gouty attacks, you certainly want the uric acid lowered. If they are free of gout, I use the drug when the uric acid gets over 9.5 or 10 mg per 100 ml.

DR. GIFFORD: I don't use it *routinely*, even if the uric acid is up to 12 or 13 mg per 100 ml. You're not worried about uric acid. I may use it when the levels are up to 10 or 12, but there are some problems with allopurinol, too, such as skin rashes, and so forth.

QUESTION: Dr. Moser, would you care to comment on Dr. Tobian's remark that patients with renovascular hypertension are extremely difficult to treat medically?

DR. MOSER: Our experience has been somewhat different. While many of them may not respond to diuretic therapy alone, we have been able to control a high percentage of patients with multiple drug therapy. This is our reason for advocating medical therapy first—in all but the specific kinds of patients Dr. Tobian and I have enumerated.

Index

D/00/5529

C I B A

Therapeutic Guide

Apresoline® hydrochloride (hydralazine hydrochloride USP)

Tablets

DESCRIPTION
Apresoline, an antihypertensive, is 1-hydrazinophthalazine monohydrochloride.

ACTIONS
Although the precise mechanism of action of Apresoline is not fully understood, the major effects are on the cardiovascular system.

Apresoline apparently lowers blood pressure by exerting a peripheral vasodilating effect through a direct relaxation of vascular smooth muscle. In both animals and man this results in: a decrease in arterial blood pressure (diastolic more than systolic); decreased peripheral vascular resistance; and an increased heart rate, stroke volume, and cardiac output. Apresoline also maintains or increases renal and cerebral blood flow.

INDICATIONS
Essential hypertension, alone or as an adjunct.

CONTRAINDICATIONS
Hypersensitivity to hydralazine; coronary artery disease; and mitral valvular rheumatic heart disease.

WARNINGS
Chronic administration of doses over 400 mg per day may produce in a few patients an arthritis-like syndrome leading to a clinical picture simulating acute systemic lupus erythematosus; this syndrome may also occur *at lower doses*. Symptoms and signs usually regress when the drug is discontinued, but long-term treatment with steroids may be necessary and residua have been detected many years later. Complete blood counts, L. E. cell preparations, and antinuclear antibody titer determinations are indicated before and periodically during prolonged therapy with hydralazine, even though the patient is asymptomatic. These studies are also indicated if the patient develops arthralgia, fever, chest pain, continued malaise, or other unexplained signs or symptoms.

Use MAO inhibitors with caution in patients receiving Apresoline.

Usage in Pregnancy
The drug should be used in pregnancy only when, in the judgment of the physician, it is deemed essential to the welfare of the patient.

PRECAUTIONS
Myocardial stimulation produced by Apresoline can cause anginal attacks and ECG changes of myocardial ischemia. The drug has been implicated in the production of myocardial infarction. It must, therefore, be used with caution in patients with suspected coronary artery disease.

The "hyperdynamic" circulation caused by Apresoline may accentuate specific cardiovascular inadequacies. An example is that Apresoline may increase pulmonary artery pressure in patients with mitral valvular disease. The drug may reduce the pressor responses to epinephrine. Postural hypotension may result from Apresoline, but is less common than with ganglionic blocking agents. Use with caution in patients with cerebral vascular accidents.

In hypertensive patients with normal kidneys who are treated with Apresoline, there is evidence of increased renal blood flow and a maintenance of glomerular filtration rate. In some instances improved renal function has been noted where control values were below normal prior to Apresoline administration. However, as with any antihypertensive agent, Apresoline should be used with caution in patients with advanced renal damage.

Peripheral neuritis, evidenced by paresthesias, numbness, and tingling, has been observed. Published evidence suggests an antipyridoxine effect and the addition of pyridoxine to the regimen if symptoms develop.

Blood dyscrasias, consisting of reduction in hemoglobin and red cell count, leukopenia, agranulocytosis, and purpura, have been reported. If such abnormalities develop, discontinue therapy. Periodic blood counts are advised during prolonged therapy.

ADVERSE REACTIONS

Adverse reactions with Apresoline are usually reversible when dosage is reduced. However, in some cases it may be necessary to discontinue the drug.

Common: Headache; palpitations; anorexia; nausea; vomiting; diarrhea; tachycardia; angina pectoris.

Less Frequent: Nasal congestion; flushing; lacrimation; conjunctivitis; peripheral neuritis, evidenced by paresthesias, numbness, and tingling; edema; dizziness; tremors; muscle cramps; psychotic reactions characterized by depression, disorientation, or anxiety; hypersensitivity (including rash, urticaria, pruritus, fever, chills, arthralgia, eosinophilia, and, rarely, hepatitis); constipation; difficulty in micturition; dyspnea; paralytic ileus; lymphadenopathy; splenomegaly; blood dyscrasias, consisting of reduction in hemoglobin and red cell count, leukopenia, agranulocytosis, and purpura; hypotension; paradoxical pressor response.

DOSAGE AND ADMINISTRATION

Initiate therapy in gradually increasing dosages; adjust according to individual response. Start with 10 mg 4 times daily for the first 2 to 4 days, increase to 25 mg 4 times daily for balance of first week. For second and subsequent weeks, increase dosage to 50 mg 4 times daily. For maintenance, adjust dosage to lowest effective levels.

The incidence of toxic reactions, particularly the L. E. cell syndrome, is high in the group of patients receiving large doses of Apresoline.

In a few resistant patients, up to 300 mg Apresoline daily may be required for a significant antihypertensive effect. In such cases, a lower dosage of Apresoline combined with a thiazide, reserpine, or both may be considered. However, when combining therapy, individual titration is essential to insure the lowest possible therapeutic dose of each drug.

OVERDOSAGE

Signs and Symptoms

Hypotension, tachycardia, headache and generalized skin flushing are to be expected. Myocardial ischemia and cardiac arrhythmia can develop; profound shock can occur in severe overdosage.

Treatment

Evacuate gastric contents, taking adequate precautions against aspiration and for protection of the airway; instill activated charcoal slurry, if general conditions permit. These manipulations may have to be omitted or carried out after cardiovascular status has been stabilized, since they might precipitate cardiac arrhythmias or increase the depth of shock.

Support of the cardiovascular system is of primary importance. Shock should be treated with volume expanders without resorting to use of vasopressors, if possible. If a vasopressor is required, use one that is least likely to precipitate or aggravate cardiac arrhythmia. Digitalization may be necessary. Renal function must be monitored and supported as required.

No experience has been reported with extracorporeal or peritoneal dialysis.

HOW SUPPLIED

Tablets, 10 mg (pale yellow, dry-coated); bottles of 30, 60, 100 and 1000.

Tablets, 25 mg (deep blue, dry-coated) and 50 mg (lilac, dry-coated); bottles of 30, 60, 100, 500 and 1000.

Tablets, 100 mg (peach, dry-coated); bottles of 100.

REV. 7/75

Apresoline® hydrochloride
(hydralazine hydrochloride USP)

Parenteral

DESCRIPTION
Apresoline, an antihypertensive, is 1-hydrazinophthalazine monohydrochloride.

ACTIONS
Although the precise mechanism of action of Apresoline is not fully understood, the major effects are on the cardiovascular system.

Apresoline apparently lowers blood pressure by exerting a peripheral vasodilating effect through a direct relaxation of vascular smooth muscle. In both animals and man this results in: a decrease in arterial blood pressure (diastolic more than systolic); decreased peripheral vascular resistance; and an increased heart rate, stroke volume, and cardiac output. Apresoline also maintains or increases renal and cerebral blood flow.

INDICATIONS
Severe essential hypertension when the drug cannot be given orally or when there is an urgent need to lower blood pressure.

CONTRAINDICATIONS
Hypersensitivity to hydralazine; coronary artery disease; and mitral valvular rheumatic heart disease.

WARNINGS
Chronic administration of doses over 400 mg per day may produce in a few patients an arthritis-like syndrome leading to a clinical picture simulating acute systemic lupus erythematosus; this syndrome may also occur *at lower doses.* Symptoms and signs usually regress when the drug is discontinued, but long-term treatment with steroids may be necessary and residua have been detected many years later. Complete blood counts, L. E. cell preparations, and antinuclear antibody titer determinations are indicated before and periodically during prolonged therapy with hydralazine, even though the patient is asymptomatic. These studies are also indicated if the patient develops arthralgia, fever, chest pain, continued malaise, or other unexplained signs or symptoms.

Use MAO inhibitors with caution in patients receiving Apresoline.

Usage in Pregnancy
The drug should be used in pregnancy only when, in the judgment of the physician, it is deemed essential to the welfare of the patient.

PRECAUTIONS
Myocardial stimulation produced by Apresoline can cause anginal attacks and ECG changes of myocardial ischemia. The drug has been implicated in the production of myocardial infarction. It must, therefore, be used with caution in patients with suspected coronary artery disease.

The "hyperdynamic" circulation caused by Apresoline may accentuate specific cardiovascular inadequacies. An example is that Apresoline may increase pulmonary artery pressure in patients with mitral valvular disease. The drug may reduce the pressor responses to epinephrine. Postural hypotension may result from Apresoline, but is less common than with ganglionic blocking agents. Use with caution in patients with cerebral vascular accidents.

In hypertensive patients with normal kidneys who are treated with Apresoline, there is evidence of increased renal blood flow and a maintenance of glomerular filtration rate. In some instances improved renal function has been noted where control values were below normal prior to Apresoline administration. However, as with any antihypertensive agent, Apresoline should be used with caution in patients with advanced renal damage.

Peripheral neuritis, evidenced by paresthesias, numbness, and tingling, has been observed. Published evidence suggests an antipyridoxine effect and the addition of pyridoxine to the regimen if symptoms develop.

Blood dyscrasias, consisting of reduction in hemoglobin and red cell count, leukopenia, agranulocytosis, and purpura, have been reported. If such abnormalities develop, discontinue therapy. Periodic blood counts are advised during prolonged therapy.

ADVERSE REACTIONS

Adverse reactions with Apresoline are usually reversible when dosage is reduced. However, in some cases it may be necessary to discontinue the drug.

Common: Headache; palpitations; anorexia; nausea; vomiting; diarrhea; tachycardia; and angina pectoris.

Less Frequent: Nasal congestion; flushing; lacrimation; conjunctivitis; peripheral neuritis, evidenced by paresthesias, numbness, and tingling; edema; dizziness; tremors; muscle cramps; psychotic reactions characterized by depression, disorientation, or anxiety; hypersensitivity (including rash, urticaria, pruritus, fever, chills, arthralgia, eosinophilia, and, rarely, hepatitis); constipation; difficulty in micturition; dyspnea; paralytic ileus; lymphadenopathy; splenomegaly; blood dyscrasias, consisting of reduction in hemoglobin and red cell count, leukopenia, agranulocytosis, and purpura; hypotension; paradoxical pressor response.

DOSAGE AND ADMINISTRATION

When there is urgent need, therapy in the hospitalized patient may be initiated intravenously or intramuscularly. Use parenteral Apresoline only when the drug cannot be given orally. Usual dose is 20 to 40 mg, repeated as necessary. Certain patients (especially those with marked renal damage) may require a lower dose. Check blood pressure frequently. It may begin to fall within a few minutes after injection, with an average maximal decrease occurring in 10 to 80 minutes. In cases where there is a previously existing increased intracranial pressure, lowering the blood pressure may increase cerebral ischemia. Most patients can be transferred to oral Apresoline within 24 to 48 hours.

OVERDOSAGE

Signs and Symptoms

Hypotension, tachycardia, headache and generalized skin flushing are to be expected. Myocardial ischemia and cardiac arrhythmia can develop; profound shock can occur in severe overdosage.

Treatment

Support of the cardiovascular system is of primary importance. Shock should be treated with volume expanders without resorting to use of vasopressors, if possible. If a vasopressor is required, use one that is least likely to precipitate or aggravate cardiac arrhythmia. Digitalization may be necessary. Renal function must be monitored and supported as required.

No experience has been reported with extracorporeal or peritoneal dialysis.

HOW SUPPLIED

Ampuls, 1 ml, each ml containing 20 mg hydralazine hydrochloride, 0.1 ml propylene glycol with 0.065% methyl-*p*-hydroxybenzoate and 0.035% propyl-*p*-hydroxybenzoate as preservatives in water; cartons of 5.

REV. 7/75

Esidrix®
(hydrochlorothiazide USP)

DESCRIPTION

Esidrix, an analog of chlorothiazide, is a white, or practically white, odorless, crystalline powder that is only slightly soluble in water. Chemically, it is 6-chloro-3,4-dihydro-2*H*-1, 2,4-benzothiadiazine-7-sulfonamide 1,1-dioxide.

ACTIONS

The mechanism of action results in an interference with the renal tubular mechanism of electrolyte reabsorption. At maximal therapeutic dosage all thiazides are approximately equal in their diuretic potency. The mechanism whereby thiazides function in the control of hypertension is unknown.

INDICATIONS

Based on a review of this drug by the National Academy of Sciences-National Research Council and/or other information, FDA has classified the indications as follows:

Effective

Hypertension: In the management of hypertension either as the sole therapeutic agent or to enhance the effect of other antihypertensive drugs in the more severe forms of hypertension.

Edema: As adjunctive therapy in edema associated with congestive heart failure, hepatic cirrhosis, and corticosteroid and estrogen therapy.

Esidrix has also been found useful in edema due to various forms of renal dysfunction, such as the nephrotic syndrome, acute glomerulonephritis, and chronic renal failure.

"Probably" Effective

Toxemia of pregnancy (eclampsia), angina due to congestive heart failure and/or hypertension, and "drug induced" edema.

Final classification of the less-than-effective indications requires further investigation.

CONTRAINDICATIONS

Anuria; hypersensitivity to this or other sulfonamide-derived drugs. The routine use of diuretics in an otherwise healthy pregnant woman with or without mild edema is contraindicated and possibly hazardous.

WARNINGS

Use with caution in severe renal disease. In patients with renal disease, thiazides may precipitate azotemia. Cumulative effects of the drug may develop in patients with impaired renal function.

Thiazides should be used with caution in patients with impaired hepatic function or progressive liver disease, since minor alterations of fluid and electrolyte imbalance may precipitate hepatic coma.

Thiazides may be additive or potentiative of the action of other antihypertensive drugs. Potentiation occurs with ganglionic or peripheral adrenergic blocking drugs.

Sensitivity reactions are more likely to occur in patients with a history of allergy or bronchial asthma.

The possibility of exacerbation or activation of systemic lupus erythematosus has been reported.

Usage in Pregnancy

Usage of thiazides in women of childbearing age requires that the potential benefits of the drug be weighed against its possible hazards to the fetus. These hazards include fetal or neonatal jaundice, thrombocytopenia, and possibly other adverse reactions which have occurred in the adult.

Nursing Mothers

Thiazides cross the placental barrier and appear in cord blood and breast milk.

PRECAUTIONS

Periodic determination of serum electrolytes to detect possible electrolyte imbalance should be performed at appropriate intervals. All patients receiving thiazide therapy should be observed for clinical signs of fluid or electrolyte imbalance: namely, hyponatremia, hypochloremic alkalosis, and hypokalemia. Serum and urine electrolyte determinations are particularly important when the patient is vomiting excessively or receiving parenteral fluids. Medication such as digitalis may also influence serum electrolytes. Warning signs are dryness of mouth, thirst, weakness, lethargy, drowsiness, restlessness, muscle pains or cramps, muscular fatigue, hypotension, oliguria, tachycardia, and gastrointestinal disturbance such as nausea or vomiting.

Hypokalemia may develop with thiazides as with any other potent diuretic, especially during brisk diuresis, when severe cirrhosis is present, or during concomitant administration of steroids or ACTH.

Interference with adequate oral intake of electrolytes will also contribute to hypokalemia. Digitalis therapy may exaggerate metabolic effects of hypokalemia especially with reference to myocardial activity.

Any chloride deficit is generally mild and usually does not require specific treatment except under extraordinary circumstances (as in liver disease or renal disease). Dilutional hyponatremia may occur in edematous patients in hot weather; appropriate therapy is water restriction, rather than administration of salt except in rare instances when the hyponatremia is life-threatening. In actual salt depletion, appropriate replacement is the therapy of choice.

Transient elevations in plasma calcium may occur in patients receiving thiazides. This may be more pronounced or sustained in patients with hyperparathyroidism. Pathological changes in the parathyroid gland have been reported in a few patients on prolonged thiazide therapy.

Hyperuricemia may occur or frank gout may be precipitated in certain patients receiving thiazide therapy.

Insulin requirements in diabetic patients may be increased, decreased, or unchanged. Latent diabetes may become manifest during thiazide administration.

Thiazide drugs may increase the responsiveness to tubocurarine.

The antihypertensive effects of the drug may be enhanced in the post-sympathectomy patient.

Thiazides may decrease arterial responsiveness to norepinephrine. This diminution is not sufficient to preclude effectiveness of the pressor agent for therapeutic use.

If progressive renal impairment becomes evident, as indicated by a rising non-protein nitrogen or blood urea nitrogen, a careful reappraisal of therapy is necessary with consideration given to withholding or discontinuing diuretic therapy.

Thiazides may decrease serum PBI levels without signs of thyroid disturbance.

ADVERSE REACTIONS

Gastrointestinal: Anorexia, gastric irritation, nausea, vomiting, cramping, diarrhea, constipation, jaundice (intrahepatic cholestatic), pancreatitis
Central Nervous System: Dizziness, vertigo, paresthesias, headache, xanthopsia
Dermatologic-Hypersensitivity: Purpura, photosensitivity, rash, urticaria, necrotizing angiitis, Stevens-Johnson syndrome, and other hypersensitivity reactions.
Hematologic: Leukopenia, agranulocytosis, thrombocytopenia, aplastic anemia
Cardiovascular: Orthostatic hypotension may occur and may be potentiated by alcohol, barbiturates, or narcotics
Other: Hyperglycemia, glycosuria, hyperuricemia, muscle spasm, weakness, restlessness

Whenever adverse reactions are moderate or severe, thiazide dosage should be reduced or therapy withdrawn.

DOSAGE AND ADMINISTRATION

Therapy should be individualized according to patient response. Dosage should be titrated to gain maximal therapeutic response as well as the minimal dose possible to maintain that therapeutic response.

Hypertension

To Initiate Therapy: Usual dose is 75 mg daily. May be given as a single dose every morning.

Maintenance: After a week dosage may be adjusted downward to as little as 25 mg a day, or upward to as much as 100 mg daily.

Combined Therapy: When necessary, other antihypertensive agents may be added cautiously. Since this drug potentiates the antihypertensive effect of other agents, such additions should be gradual. Dosages of ganglionic blockers in particular should be halved initially.

Edema

To Initiate Diuresis: 25 to 200 mg daily for several days, or until dry weight is attained.

Maintenance: 25 to 100 mg daily or intermittently depending on patient's response. A few refractory patients may require up to 200 mg daily.

OVERDOSAGE

Signs and Symptoms

Diuresis is to be expected; lethargy of varying degree may appear and may progress to coma within a few hours, with minimal depression of respiration and cardiovascular function and without significant serum electrolyte changes or dehydration. The mechanism of CNS depression with thiazide overdosage is unknown.

GI irritation and hypermotility may occur; temporary elevation of BUN has been reported and serum electrolyte changes could occur, especially in patients with impairment of renal function.

Treatment

Evacuate gastric contents but take care to prevent aspiration, especially in the stuporous or comatose patient. GI effects are usually of short duration, but may require symptomatic treatment.

Monitor serum electrolyte levels and renal function; institute supportive measures as required individually to maintain hydration, electrolyte balance, respiration and cardio-vascular-renal function.

HOW SUPPLIED

Tablets, 50 mg (yellow, scored); bottles of 30, 60, 100, 1000, 5000 and Accu-Pak® blister units of 100.
Tablets, 25 mg (pink, scored); bottles of 30, 60, 100, 1000 and 5000.

REV. 6/75

Gammacorten®
(dexamethasone USP)

DESCRIPTION

Gammacorten, the 9-alpha fluoro, 16-alpha methyl derivative of prednisolone, is a potent glucocorticoid.

Glucocorticoids are adrenocortical steroids, both naturally occurring and synthetic, which are readily absorbed from the gastro-intestinal tract.

ACTIONS

Naturally occurring glucocorticoids (hydro-cortisone and cortisone), which also have salt-retaining properties, are used as replacement therapy in adrenocortical deficiency states. Their synthetic analogs are primarily used for their potent anti-inflammatory effects in disorders of many organ systems.

Glucocorticoids cause profound and varied metabolic effects. In addition, they modify the body's immune responses to diverse stimuli.

INDICATIONS

Based on a review of this drug by the National Academy of Sciences-National Research Council and/or other information, FDA has classified the indications as follows:

Effective

Endocrine Disorders: Primary or secondary adrenocortical insufficiency (hydrocortisone or cortisone is the first choice; synthetic analogs may be used in conjunction with mineralocorticoids where applicable; in infancy mineralo-corticoid supplementation is of particular importance); congenital adrenal hyperplasia; nonsuppurative thyroiditis; hypercalcemia associated with cancer.

Rheumatic Disorders: As adjunctive therapy for short-term administration (to tide the patient over an acute episode or exacerbation) in psoriatic arthritis, rheumatoid arthritis (selected cases may require low-dose maintenance therapy), ankylosing spondylitis, acute and subacute bursitis, acute nonspecific tenosynovitis, acute gouty arthritis.

Collagen Diseases: During an exacerbation or as maintenance therapy in selected cases of systemic lupus erythematosus and acute rheumatic carditis.

Dermatologic Diseases: Pemphigus, bullous dermatitis herpetiformis, severe erythema multiforme (Stevens-Johnson syndrome), exfoliative dermatitis, mycosis fungoides, severe psoriasis.

Allergic States: Control of severe or incapacitating allergic conditions intractable to adequate trials of conventional treatment: Seasonal or perennial allergic rhinitis, bronchial asthma, contact dermatitis, atopic dermatitis, serum sickness.

Ophthalmic Diseases: Severe acute and chronic allergic and inflammatory processes involving the eye and its adnexa: Allergic conjunctivitis, keratitis, allergic corneal marginal ulcers, herpes zoster ophthalmicus, iritis and iridocyclitis, chorioretinitis, anterior segment inflammation, diffuse posterior uveitis and choroiditis, optic neuritis, sympathetic ophthalmia.

Respiratory Diseases: Symptomatic sarcoidosis, Loeffler's syndrome not manageable by other means, berylliosis, fulminating or disseminated pulmonary tuberculosis when concurrently accompanied by appropriate antituberculous chemotherapy.

Hematologic Disorders: Idiopathic and secondary thrombocytopenia in adults, acquired (autoimmune) hemolytic anemia, erythroblastopenia (RBC anemia), congenital (erythroid) hypoplastic anemia.

Neoplastic Diseases: For palliative management of leukemias and lymphomas in adults and acute leukemia of childhood.

Edematous States: To induce a diuresis or remission of proteinuria in the nephrotic syndrome, without uremia, of the idiopathic type or that due to lupus erythematosus.

Miscellaneous: Tuberculous meningitis with subarachnoid block or impending block when concurrently accompanied by appropriate antituberculous chemotherapy and diagnostic testing of adrenocortical hyperfunction.

"Probably" effective

Allergic States: Control of severe or incapacitating angio-edema or urticaria intractable to adequate trials of conventional treatment.

Respiratory Diseases: Pulmonary emphysema where bronchospasm or bronchial edema plays a significant role; diffuse interstitial pulmonary fibrosis (Hamman-Rich syndrome).

Edematous States: In conjunction with diuretic agents, to induce diuresis in cirrhosis of the liver with refractory ascites and in refractory congestive heart failure.

Gastrointestinal Diseases: To tide the patient over a critical period of the disease in ulcerative colitis, regional enteritis, and intractable sprue.

Miscellaneous: Dental postoperative inflammatory reactions.

Final classification of the less-than-effective indications requires further investigation.

CONTRAINDICATIONS

Systemic fungal infections.

WARNINGS

In patients on corticosteroid therapy subjected to unusual stress, increased dosage of rapidly acting corticosteroids before, during, and after the stressful situation is indicated.

Corticosteroids may mask some signs of infection, and new infections may appear during their use. There may be decreased resistance and inability to localize infection when corticosteroids are used.

Prolonged use of corticosteroids may produce posterior subcapsular cataracts, glaucoma with possible damage to the optic nerves, and may enhance the establishment of secondary ocular infections due to fungi or viruses.

Average and large doses of hydrocortisone or cortisone can cause elevation of blood pressure, salt and water retention, and increased excretion of potassium. These effects are less likely to occur with the synthetic derivatives except when used in large doses. Dietary salt restriction and potassium supplementation may be necessary. All corticosteriods increase calcium excretion.

While on corticosteroid therapy patients should not be vaccinated against smallpox. Other immunization procedures should not be undertaken in patients who are on corticosteroids, especially on high dose, because of possible hazards of neurological complications and a lack of antibody response.

The use of Gammacorten in active tuberculosis should be restricted to those cases of fulminating or disseminated tuberculosis in which the corticosteroid is used for the management of the disease in conjunction with an appropriate antituberculous regimen.

If corticosteroids are indicated in patients with latent tuberculosis or tuberculin reactivity, close observation is necessary as reactivation of the disease may occur. During prolonged corticosteroid therapy these patients should receive chemoprophylaxis.

Usage in Pregnancy

Since adequate human reproduction studies have not been done with corticosteroids, the use of these drugs in pregnancy, nursing mothers or women of childbearing potential requires that the possible benefits of the drug be weighed against the potential hazards to the mother and embryo or fetus. Infants born of mothers who have received substantial doses of corticosteroids during pregnancy should be carefully observed for signs of hypoadrenalism.

Drug Interactions

Anticonvulsant drugs may cause an acceleration of the hepatic conjugation and biliary excretion of dexamethasone. This may lead to lower blood levels of free dexamethasone or its metabolites and less inhibition of ACTH secretion.

PRECAUTIONS

Drug-induced secondary adrenocortical insufficiency may be minimized by gradual reduction of dosage. This type of relative insufficiency may persist for months after discontinuation of therapy; therefore, in any situation of stress occurring during that period, hormone therapy should be reinstituted. Since mineralocorticoid secretion may be impaired, salt and/or a mineralocorticoid should be administered concurrently.

There is an enhanced effect of corticosteroids in patients with hypothyroidism and in those with cirrhosis.

Corticosteroids should be used cautiously in patients with ocular herpes simplex because of possible corneal perforation.

The lowest possible dose of corticosteroid should be used to control the condition under treatment, and when reduction in dosage is possible, the reduction should be gradual.

Psychic derangements may appear when corticosteroids are used, ranging from euphoria, insomnia, mood swings, personality changes, and severe depression, to frank psychotic manifestations. Also, existing emotional instability or psychotic tendencies may be aggravated by corticosteroids.

Aspirin should be used cautiously in conjunction with corticosteroids in hypoprothrombinemia.

Steroids should be used with caution: in nonspecific ulcerative colitis, if there is a probability of impending perforation, abscess or other pyogenic infection; diverticulitis; fresh intestinal anastomoses; active or latent peptic ulcer; renal insufficiency; hypertension; osteoporosis; and myasthenia gravis.

Growth and development of infants and children on prolonged corticosteroid therapy should be carefully observed.

ADVERSE REACTIONS

Fluid and Electrolyte Disturbances: Sodium retention; fluid retention; congestive heart failure in susceptible patients; potassium loss; hypokalemic alkalosis; hypertension.

Musculoskeletal: Muscle weakness; steroid myopathy; loss of muscle mass; osteoporosis; vertebral compression fractures; aseptic necrosis of femoral and humeral heads; pathologic fracture of long bones.

Gastrointestinal: Peptic ulcer with possible perforation and hemorrhage; pancreatitis; abdominal distention; ulcerative esophagitis.

Dermatologic: Impaired wound healing; thin fragile skin; petechiae and ecchymoses; facial erythema; increased sweating; may suppress reactions to skin tests.

Neurological: Convulsions; increased intracranial pressure with papilledema (pseudotumor cerebri), usually after treatment; vertigo; headache.

Endocrine: Menstrual irregularities; development of Cushingoid state; suppression of growth in children; secondary adrenocortical and pituitary unresponsiveness, particularly in times of stress as in trauma, surgery, or illness; decreased carbohydrate tolerance; manifestations of latent diabetes mellitus; increased requirements for insulin or oral hypoglycemic agents in diabetics.

Ophthalmic: Posterior subcapsular cataracts; increased intraocular pressure; glaucoma; exophthalmos.

Metabolic: Negative nitrogen balance due to protein catabolism.

DOSAGE AND ADMINISTRATION

The initial dosage of Gammacorten may vary from 0.75 mg. to 9.0 mg per day depending on the specific disease entity being treated. In situations of less severity, lower doses will generally suffice while in selected patients, higher initial doses may be required. The initial dosage should be maintained or adjusted until a satisfactory response is noted. If after a reasonable period of time there is a lack of satisfactory clinical response, Gammacorten should be discontinued and the patient transferred to other appropriate therapy.

IT SHOULD BE EMPHASIZED THAT DOSAGE REQUIREMENTS ARE VARIABLE AND MUST BE INDIVIDUALIZED ON THE BASIS OF THE DISEASE UNDER TREATMENT AND THE RESPONSE OF THE PATIENT.

After a favorable response is noted, the proper maintenance dosage should be determined by decreasing the initial drug dosage in small increments at appropriate time intervals until the lowest dosage which will maintain an adequate clinical response is reached.

It should be kept in mind that constant monitoring is needed in regard to drug dosage. Included in the situations which may make dosage adjustments necessary are changes in clinical status secondary to remissions or exacerbations in the disease process, the patient's individual drug responsiveness, and the effect of patient exposure to stressful situations not directly related to the disease entity under treatment; in this latter situation it may be necessary to increase the dosage of Gammacorten for a period of time consistent with the patient's condition. If after long-term therapy the drug is to be stopped, it is recommended that it be withdrawn gradually rather than abruptly.

HOW SUPPLIED

Tablets, 0.75 mg (bluish pink, scored); bottles of 250.

REV. 3/72

Ismelin® sulfate
(guanethidine sulfate USP)

DESCRIPTION
Guanethidine is a white crystalline powder that is very soluble in water and practically insoluble in chloroform. Chemically, it is [2-(hexahydro-1(2*H*)-azocinyl) ethyl]-guanidine sulfate.

ACTIONS
Pharmacologically, guanethidine inhibits or interferes with the release and/or distribution of the chemical mediator (presumably the catecholamine, norepinephrine) at the sympathetic neuroeffector junction. In contrast to ganglionic blocking agents, Ismelin suppresses equally the responses mediated by *alpha* and *beta* adrenergic receptors but does not produce parasympathetic blockade. Since sympathetic blockade results in modest decreases in peripheral resistance and cardiac output, Ismelin lowers blood pressure in the supine position. It further reduces blood pressure by decreasing the degree of vasoconstriction which normally results from reflex sympathetic nervous activity on assumption of the upright posture, thus reducing the venous return and cardiac output more. The inhibition of sympathetic venoconstrictive mechanisms results in venous pooling of blood. Therefore, the effect of Ismelin is especially pronounced when the patient is standing. Both the systolic and diastolic pressures are reduced.

INDICATIONS
Moderate and severe hypertension either alone or as an adjunct.
Renal hypertension, including that secondary to pyelonephritis, renal amyloidosis, and renal artery stenosis.

CONTRAINDICATIONS
Known or suspected pheochromocytoma; hypersensitivity; frank congestive heart failure not due to hypertension; use of MAO inhibitors.

WARNINGS
Ismelin is a potent drug and can lead to disturbing and serious clinical problems. Before prescribing, physicians should familiarize themselves with the details of its use and warn patients not to deviate from instructions.

> Orthostatic hypotension can occur frequently and patients should be properly instructed about this potential hazard. Fainting spells may occur unless the patient is forewarned to sit or lie down with the onset of dizziness or weakness. Postural hypotension is most marked in the morning and is accentuated by hot weather, alcohol, or exercise. Dizziness or weakness may be particularly bothersome during the initial period of dosage adjustment and with postural changes, such as arising in the morning. The potential occurrence of these symptoms may require alteration of previous daily activity. The patient should be cautioned to avoid sudden or prolonged standing or exercise while taking the drug.

Concurrent use of Ismelin and rauwolfia derivatives may cause excessive postural hypotension, bradycardia, and mental depression.

If possible, withdraw therapy two weeks prior to surgery to reduce the possibility of vascular collapse and cardiac arrest during anesthesia. If emergency surgery is indicated, preanesthetic and anesthetic agents should be administered cautiously in reduced dosage. Oxygen, atropine, vasopressors, and adequate solutions for volume replacement should be ready for immediate use to counteract vascular collapse in the surgical patient. Vasopressors should be used only with extreme caution, since Ismelin augments the responsiveness to exogenously administered norepinephrine and vasopressors with respect to blood pressure and their propensity for the production of cardiac arrhythmias.

Dosage requirements may be reduced in

the presence of fever.

Exercise special care when treating patients with a history of bronchial asthma; asthmatics are more apt to be hypersensitive to catecholamine depletion and their condition may be aggravated.

Usage in Pregnancy

The safety of Ismelin for use in pregnancy has not been established; therefore this drug should be used in pregnant patients only when, in the judgment of the physician, its use is deemed essential to the welfare of the patient.

PRECAUTIONS

The effects of guanethidine are cumulative over long periods; initial doses should be small and increased gradually in small increments.

Use very cautiously in hypertensive patients with: renal disease and nitrogen retention or rising BUN levels, since decreased blood pressure may further compromise renal function; coronary disease with insufficiency or recent myocardial infarction; cerebral vascular disease, especially with encephalopathy.

Do not give to patients with severe cardiac failure except with extreme caution since Ismelin may interfere with the compensatory role of the adrenergic system in producing circulatory adjustment in patients with congestive heart failure.

In patients with incipient cardiac decompensation, watch for weight gain or edema, which may be averted by the concomitant administration of a thiazide.

Remember that both digitalis and Ismelin slow the heart rate.

Use cautiously in patients with a history of peptic ulcer or other chronic disorders which may be aggravated by a relative increase in parasympathetic tone.

Amphetamine-like compounds, stimulants (*eg*, ephedrine, methylphenidate), tricyclic antidepressants (*eg*, amitriptyline, imipramine, desipramine) and other psychopharmacologic agents (*eg*, phenothiazines and related compounds), and oral contraceptives may reduce the hypotensive effect of guanethidine.

MAO inhibitors should be discontinued for at least one week before starting therapy with Ismelin.

ADVERSE REACTIONS

Frequent reactions due to sympathetic blockade: dizziness, weakness, lassitude, and syncope resulting from either postural or exertional hypotension.

Frequent reactions due to unopposed parasympathetic activity: bradycardia, increase in bowel movements, and diarrhea. Diarrhea may be severe at times and necessitate discontinuance of the medication.

Other common reactions: inhibition of ejaculation, a tendency toward fluid retention and edema with occasional development of congestive heart failure.

Other less common reactions: dyspnea, fatigue, nausea, vomiting, nocturia, urinary incontinence, dermatitis, scalp hair loss, dry mouth, rise in BUN, ptosis of the lids, blurring of vision, parotid tenderness, myalgia, muscle tremor, mental depression, chest pains (angina), chest paresthesias, nasal congestion, weight gain, and asthma in susceptible individuals. Although a causal relationship has not been established, a few instances of anemia, thrombocytopenia and leukopenia have been reported.

DOSAGE AND ADMINISTRATION

Better control may be obtained, especially in the initial phases of treatment, if the patient can have his blood pressure recorded regularly at home.

Ambulatory Patients. Begin treatment with small doses (10 mg). Increase gradually, depending upon the patient's response. Ismelin has a long duration of action; therefore, dosage increases should not be made more often than every 5 to 7 days, unless the patient is hospitalized.

Take blood pressure in the supine position, after standing for ten minutes, and immediately after exercise if feasible. Increase dosage only if there has been *no* decrease in standing blood pressure from the previous levels. The average daily dose is 25 to 50 mg; only 1 dose a day is usually required.

Dosage Chart for Ambulatory Patients

Visits at Intervals of 5 to 7 Days	*Daily Dose*
Visit No. 1 (Start with 10-mg tablets)	10 mg
Visit No. 2	20 mg
Visit No. 3 (Patient can be changed to 25-mg tablets whenever convenient)	30 mg (three 10-mg tablets) or 37.5 mg (one and one-half 25-mg tablets)
Visit No. 4	50 mg
Visit No. 5 (and subsequent). Dosage may be increased by 12.5 mg or 25 mg if necessary.	

Reduce dosage in any of the following 3 situations:

1. *Normal supine pressure*
2. *Excessive orthostatic fall in pressure*
3. *Severe diarrhea*

Hospitalized Patients. Initial oral dose is 25 to 50 mg, increased by 25 or 50 mg daily or every other day as indicated. This higher dosage is possible because hospitalized patients can be watched carefully. Unless absolutely impossible, take the standing blood pressure regularly. Patients should not be discharged from the hospital until the effect of the drug on the standing blood pressure is known. *Patients should be told about the possibility of orthostatic hypotension and warned not to get out of bed without help during the period of dosage adjustment.*

Combination Therapy. Ismelin may be added gradually to thiazides and/or hydralazine. Thiazide diuretics enhance the effectiveness of Ismelin and may reduce the incidence of edema. When thiazide diuretics are added to the regimen in patients on Ismelin, it is usually necessary to reduce the dosage of Ismelin. After control is established, reduce dosage of all drugs to the lowest effective level.

When replacing MAO inhibitors, at least one week should elapse before commencing treatment with Ismelin.

In many cases ganglionic blockers will have been stopped before Ismelin is started. It may be advisable, however, to withdraw the blocker gradually to prevent a spiking blood pressure response during the transfer period.

OVERDOSAGE

Signs and Symptoms

Postural hypotension [with dizziness, blurring of vision, etc., possibly progressing to syncope when standing] and bradycardia are most likely to occur; diarrhea, possibly severe, also may occur. Unconsciousness is unlikely if adequate blood pressure and cerebral perfusion can be maintained by appropriate positioning [supine] and by other treatment as required.

Treatment

In previously normotensive patients, treatment has consisted essentially of restoring blood pressure and heart rate to normal by keeping patient in supine position. Normal homeostatic control usually returns gradually over a 72-hour period in these patients.

In previously hypertensive patients, particularly those with impaired cardiac reserve or other cardiovascular-renal disease, intensive treatment may be required to support vital functions and/or to control cardiac irregularities that might be present. Supine position must be maintained; if vasopressors are required, it must be remembered that Ismelin may increase responsiveness as to blood pressure rise and occurrence of cardiac arrhythmias.

Diarrhea, if severe or persistent, should be treated symptomatically to reduce intestinal hypermotility, with due attention to maintenance of hydration and electrolyte balance.

HOW SUPPLIED

Tablets, 10 mg (pale yellow, scored) and 25 mg (white, scored); bottles of 30, 60, 100 and 1000.

REV. 10/74

Regitine®
(phentolamine)

DESCRIPTION
Regitine is *m*-[N-(2-Imidazolin-2-ylmethyl)-p-toluidino] phenol. The lyophilized form for injection is the methanesulfonate (mesylate) salt, and the tablet form for oral use is the hydrochloride salt.

ACTIONS
Regitine produces an alpha adrenergic block of relatively short duration. It also has direct but less marked positive inotropic and chronotropic effects on cardiac muscle and vasodilator effects on vascular smooth muscle.

INDICATIONS
Oral and Parenteral Regitine
Prevention or control of hypertensive episodes that may occur in a patient with pheochromocytoma as a result of stress or manipulation during preoperative preparation and surgical excision.

Parenteral Regitine
Prevention and treatment of dermal necrosis and sloughing following intravenous administration or extravasation of norepinephrine.

Diagnosis of pheochromocytoma—Regitine blocking test.

CONTRAINDICATIONS
Myocardial infarction, history of myocardial infarction, coronary insufficiency, angina or other evidence suggestive of coronary artery disease. Hypersensitivity to phentolamine or related compounds.

WARNINGS
Myocardial infarction, cerebrovascular spasm, and cerebrovascular occlusion have been reported to occur following the administration of phentolamine, usually in association with marked hypotensive episodes with shock-like states which occasionally follow parenteral administration.

For screening tests in patients with hypertension, the generally available urinary assay of catecholamines or other biochemical assays have largely supplanted the Regitine and other pharmacological tests for reasons of accuracy and safety. None of the chemical or pharmacological tests is infallible in the diagnosis of pheochromocytoma. The Regitine test is not the procedure of choice and should be reserved for cases in which additional confirmatory evidence is necessary, and the relative risks involved in conducting the test have been considered.

Usage in Pregnancy
The safe use of this drug in pregnant women or during lactation has not been established. Therefore, the benefits must be weighed against the potential hazards.

PRECAUTIONS
Tachycardia and cardiac arrhythmias may occur with the use of Regitine or other alpha adrenergic blocking agents. When possible, defer administration of cardiac glycosides until cardiac rhythm returns to normal.

ADVERSE REACTIONS
Acute and prolonged hypotensive episodes, tachycardia, and cardiac arrhythmias have been reported, most frequently after parenteral administration. In addition, weakness, dizziness, flushing, orthostatic hypotension, nasal stuffiness, nausea, vomiting, and diarrhea may occur.

DOSAGE AND ADMINISTRATION
1. **Prevention or control of hypertensive episodes in the patient with pheochromocytoma.**

To control and prevent paroxysmal attacks prior to surgery, the usual adult dosage is 50 mg (1 tablet) of Regitine hydrochloride orally 4 to 6 times daily. In certain severe cases, higher doses may be required. In children, smaller doses generally suffice; 25 mg (½ tablet) orally 4 to 6 times daily is suggested initially.

For use in preoperative reduction of elevated blood pressure, inject 5 mg of Regitine mesylate (1 mg for children) intravenously or intramuscularly 1 or 2 hours before surgery (and repeat if necessary).

During surgery administer Regitine mesylate (5 mg for adults, 1 mg for children) intravenously as indicated to help prevent or control paroxysms of hypertension, tachycardia, respiratory depression, convulsions, or other effects of epinephrine intoxication. (Postoperatively, norepinephrine may be given to control the hypotension which commonly follows complete removal of a pheochromocytoma.)

2. **Prevention and treatment of dermal necrosis and sloughing following intravenous administration or extravasation of norepinephrine.**

For prevention, add 10 mg Regitine mesylate to each liter of solution containing norepinephrine. The pressor effect of norepinephrine is not affected.
For treatment, inject Regitine mesylate (5 to 10 mg in 10 ml saline) into the area of extravasation within 12 hours.

3. **Diagnosis of pheochromocytoma— Regitine blocking test.**

   a. **Intravenous**
   Preparation
   Review the *Contraindications, Warnings,* and *Precautions.* Withhold sedatives, analgesics, and all other medication not deemed essential (such as digitalis and insulin) for at least 24 hours (preferably 48 to 72 hours) prior to the test. Withhold antihypertensive drugs until blood pressure returns to the untreated, hypertensive level. Do not perform test on a patient who is normotensive.

Procedure

1. Keep patient at rest in the supine position throughout the test, preferably in a quiet, darkened room. Delay Regitine injection until blood pressure is stabilized, as evidenced by blood pressure readings taken every 10 minutes for at least one-half hour.
2. Dissolve 5 mg Regitine mesylate in 1 ml Sterile Water for Injection. Dose for adults is 5 mg; for children, 1 mg.
3. Insert the syringe needle into vein, delay injection until pressor response to venipuncture has subsided.
4. Inject Regitine rapidly. Record blood pressure immediately after injection, at 30-second intervals for the first 3 minutes, and at 60-second intervals for the next 7 minutes.

Interpreting the Test
Positive response, suggestive of pheochromocytoma, is indicated by a drop in blood pressure of more than 35 mm Hg systolic and 25 mm Hg diastolic pressure. A typical positive response may be a drop of 60 mm Hg systolic and 25 mm Hg diastolic. Maximal depressor pressure effect usually is evident within 2 minutes after injection. Return to pre-injection pressure commonly occurs within 15 to 30 minutes, but may return more rapidly.

If blood pressure falls to a dangerous level, treat patient as outlined under "Overdosage."

A positive response should always be confirmed by other diagnostic procedures, preferably the measurement of urinary catecholamines or their metabolites.

Negative response is indicated when the blood pressure is unchanged, elevated, or is reduced less than 35 mm Hg systolic and 25 mm Hg diastolic after injection of Regitine. A negative response to this test does not exclude the diagnosis of pheochromocytoma, especially in patients with paroxysmal hypertension in whom the incidence of false negative responses is high.

b. **Intramuscular**

If the intramuscular test for pheochromocytoma is preferred, preparation is the same as for the intravenous test. Then dissolve 5 mg Regitine mesylate in 1 ml Sterile Water for Injection. Dose for adults is 5 mg intramuscularly; for children, 3 mg. Record blood pressure every 5 minutes for 30 to 45 minutes following intramuscular injection. Positive response is indicated by a drop in blood pressure of 35 mm Hg systolic and 25 mm Hg diastolic or greater within 20 minutes following injection.

c. **Reliability**

The test is most reliable in detecting pheochromocytoma in patients with sustained hypertension, and least reliable in those with paroxysmal hypertension. False positive tests may occur in patients with hypertension without pheochromocytoma.

OVERDOSAGE
In the event of a drop in blood pressure to dangerous level or other evidence of shock-like conditions, treat vigorously and promptly. Include intravenous infusion of norepinephrine, titrated to maintain blood pressure to normotensive level, and all available supportive measures. Do not use epinephrine since it may cause a paradoxical fall in blood pressure.

HOW SUPPLIED
Ampuls, each containing 5 mg phentolamine mesylate USP and 5 mg lactose in lyophilized form and accompanied by ampul containing 1 ml Sterile Water for Injection; cartons of 1, boxes of 6 cartons.
Tablets (white, scored), each containing 50 mg phentolamine hydrochloride NF; bottles of 100.
REV. 7/75

Ser-Ap-Es®

reserpine	**0.1 mg**
hydralazine hydrochloride	**25 mg**
hydrochlorothiazide	**15 mg**

Combination Tablets

WARNING
This fixed combination drug is not indicated for initial therapy of hypertension. Hypertension requires therapy titrated to the individual patient. If the fixed combination represents the dosage so determined, its use may be more convenient in patient management. The treatment of hypertension is not static, but must be reevaluated as conditions in each patient warrant.

DESCRIPTION
Ser-Ap-Es is a diuretic-antihypertensive combination containing: (1) reserpine, a pure crystalline alkaloid of rauwolfia; (2) hydralazine hydrochloride, an antihypertensive; and (3) hydrochlorothiazide, an analog of chlorothiazide having antihypertensive and diuretic effects.

Reserpine is methyl-O-(3,4,5-trimethoxybenzoyl)-reserpate.

Hydralazine hydrochloride is 1-hydrazinophthalazine monohydrochloride.

Hydrochlorothiazide is 6-chloro-3,4-dihydro-2*H*-1,2,4-benzothiadiazine-7-sulfonamide 1,1-dioxide.

ACTIONS

Reserpine
Reserpine probably produces its antihypertensive effects through depletion of tissue stores of catecholamines (epinephrine and norepinephrine) from peripheral sites. This depression of sympathetic nerve function results in a decreased heart rate and a lowering of arterial blood pressure. In contrast, its sedative and tranquilizing properties are thought to be related to depletion of 5-hydroxytryptamine from the brain.

Reserpine, like other rauwolfia compounds, is characterized by slow onset of action and sustained effects. Both cardiovascular and central nervous system effects may persist for a period of time following withdrawal of the drug.

Hydralazine
Although the precise mechanism of action of hydralazine is not fully understood, the major effects are on the cardiovascular system.

Hydralazine apparently lowers blood pressure by exerting a peripheral vasodilating effect through a direct relaxation of vascular smooth muscle. In both animals and man this results in: a decrease in arterial blood pressure (diastolic more than systolic); decreased peripheral vascular resistance; and an increased heart rate, stroke volume, and cardiac output. Hydralazine also maintains or increases renal and cerebral blood flow.

Hydrochlorothiazide

The mechanism of action results in an interference with the renal tubular mechanism of electrolyte reabsorption. At maximal therapeutic dosage all thiazides are approximately equal in their diuretic potency. The mechanism whereby thiazides function in the control of hypertension is unknown.

INDICATIONS

Hypertension. (See box warning.)

CONTRAINDICATIONS

Reserpine

Known hypersensitivity, mental depression (especially with suicidal tendencies), active peptic ulcer, ulcerative colitis, and patients receiving electroconvulsive therapy.

Hydralazine

Hypersensitivity to hydralazine; coronary artery disease; and mitral valvular rheumatic heart disease.

Hydrochlorothiazide

Anuria; hypersensitivity to this or other sulfonamide-derived drugs. The routine use of diuretics in an otherwise healthy pregnant woman with or without mild edema is contraindicated and possibly hazardous.

WARNINGS

Reserpine

Extreme caution should be exercised in treating patients with a history of mental depression. Discontinue the drug at first sign of despondency, early morning insomnia, loss of appetite, impotence, or self-deprecation. Drug-induced depression may persist for several months after drug withdrawal and may be severe enough to result in suicide.

MAO inhibitors should be avoided or used with extreme caution.

Hydralazine

Chronic administration of doses over 400 mg per day may produce in a few patients an arthritis-like syndrome leading to a clinical picture simulating acute systemic lupus erythematosus; this syndrome may also occur *at lower doses.* Symptoms and signs usually regress when the drug is discontinued, but long-term treatment with steroids may be necessary and residua have been detected many years later. Complete blood counts, L. E. cell preparations, and antinuclear antibody titer determinations are indicated before and periodically during prolonged therapy with hydralazine, even though the patient is asymptomatic. These studies are also indicated if the patient develops arthralgia, fever, chest pain, continued malaise, or other unexplained signs or symptoms.

Use MAO inhibitors with caution in patients receiving hydralazine.

Hydrochlorothiazide

Use with caution in severe renal disease. In patients with renal disease, thiazides may precipitate azotemia. Cumulative effects of the drug may develop in patients with impaired renal function.

Thiazides should be used with caution in patients with impaired hepatic function or progressive liver disease, since minor alterations of fluid and electrolyte imbalance may precipitate hepatic coma.

Thiazides may be additive or potentiative of the action of other antihypertensive drugs. Potentiation occurs with ganglionic or peripheral adrenergic blocking drugs.

Sensitivity reactions are more likely to occur in patients with a history of allergy or bronchial asthma.

The possibility of exacerbation or activation of systemic lupus erythematosus has been reported.

Usage in Pregnancy

Reserpine

The safety of reserpine for use during pregnancy or lactation has not been established; therefore, the drug should be used in pregnant patients or in women of childbearing potential only when, in the judgment of the physician, it is essential to the welfare of the patient. Increased respiratory tract secretions, nasal congestion, cyanosis, and anorexia may occur in neonates and breast-fed infants of reserpine-treated mothers since reserpine crosses the placental barrier and appears in maternal breast milk.

Hydralazine
The drug should be used in pregnancy only when, in the judgment of the physician, it is deemed essential to the welfare of the patient.

Hydrochlorothiazide
Usage of thiazides in women of childbearing age requires that the potential benefits of the drug be weighed against its possible hazards to the fetus. These hazards include fetal or neonatal jaundice, thrombocytopenia, and possibly other adverse reactions which have occurred in the adult.

Nursing Mothers
Thiazides cross the placental barrier and appear in cord blood and breast milk.

PRECAUTIONS

Reserpine
Since reserpine increases gastrointestinal motility and secretion, it should be used cautiously in patients with a history of peptic ulcer, ulcerative colitis, or gallstones (biliary colic may be precipitated).

Caution should be exercised when treating hypertensive patients with renal insufficiency since they adjust poorly to lowered blood pressure levels.

Use reserpine cautiously with digitalis and quinidine, since cardiac arrhythmias have occurred with rauwolfia preparations.

Preoperative withdrawal of reserpine does not assure that circulatory instability will not occur. It is important that the anesthesiologist be aware of the patient's drug intake and consider this in the overall management, since hypotension has occurred in patients receiving rauwolfia preparations. Anticholinergic and/or adrenergic drugs (*eg*, metaraminol, norepinephrine) have been employed to treat adverse vagocirculatory effects.

Hydralazine
Myocardial stimulation produced by hydralazine can cause anginal attacks and ECG changes of myocardial ischemia. The drug has been implicated in the production of myocardial infarction. It must, therefore, be used with caution in patients with suspected coronary artery disease.

The "hyperdynamic" circulation caused by hydralazine may accentuate specific cardiovascular inadequacies. An example is that hydralazine may increase pulmonary artery pressure in patients with mitral valvular disease. The drug may reduce the pressor responses to epinephrine. Postural hypotension may result from hydralazine but is less common than with ganglionic blocking agents. Use with caution in patients with cerebral vascular accidents.

In hypertensive patients with normal kidneys who are treated with hydralazine, there is evidence of increased renal blood flow and a maintenance of glomerular filtration rate. In some instances improved renal function has been noted where control values were below normal prior to hydralazine administration. However, as with any antihypertensive agent, hydralazine should be used with caution in patients with advanced renal damage.

Peripheral neuritis, evidenced by paresthesias, numbness, and tingling, has been observed. Published evidence suggests an antipyridoxine effect and the addition of pyridoxine to the regimen if symptoms develop.

Blood dyscrasias, consisting of reduction in hemoglobin and red cell count, leukopenia, agranulocytosis, and purpura, have been reported. If such abnormalities develop, discontinue therapy. Periodic blood counts are advised during prolonged therapy.

Hydrochlorothiazide
Periodic determination of serum electrolytes to detect possible electrolyte imbalance should be performed at appropriate intervals. All patients receiving thiazide therapy should be observed for clinical signs of fluid or electrolyte imbalance; namely, hyponatremia, hypochloremic alkalosis, and hypokalemia. Serum and urine electrolyte determinations are particularly important when the patient is vomiting excessively or receiving parenteral fluids. Medication such as digitalis may also influence serum electrolytes. Warning signs are dryness of mouth, thirst, weakness, lethargy, drowsiness, restlessness, muscle pains or cramps, muscular fatigue, hypotension, oliguria, tachycardia, and gastrointestinal

disturbance such as nausea or vomiting.

Hypokalemia may develop with thiazides as with any other potent diuretic, especially during brisk diuresis, when severe cirrhosis is present, or during concomitant administration of steroids or ACTH.

Interference with adequate oral intake of electrolytes will also contribute to hypokalemia. Digitalis therapy may exaggerate metabolic effects of hypokalemia especially with reference to myocardial activity.

Any chloride deficit is generally mild and usually does not require specific treatment except under extraordinary circumstances (as in liver disease or renal disease). Dilutional hyponatremia may occur in edematous patients in hot weather; appropriate therapy is water restriction rather than administration of salt, except in rare instances when the hyponatremia is life-threatening. In actual salt depletion, appropriate replacement is the therapy of choice.

Transient elevations in plasma calcium may occur in patients receiving thiazides. This may be more pronounced or sustained in patients with hyperparathyroidism. Pathological changes in the parathyroid gland have been reported in a few patients on prolonged thiazide therapy.

Hyperuricemia may occur or frank gout may be precipitated in certain patients receiving thiazide therapy.

Insulin requirements in diabetic patients may be increased, decreased, or unchanged. Latent diabetes may become manifest during thiazide administration.

Thiazide drugs may increase the responsiveness to tubocurarine.

The antihypertensive effects of the drug may be enhanced in the post-sympathectomy patient.

Thiazides may decrease arterial responsiveness to norepinephrine. This diminution is not sufficient to preclude effectiveness of the pressor agent for therapeutic use.

If progressive renal impairment becomes evident, as indicated by a rising non-protein nitrogen or blood urea nitrogen, a careful reappraisal of therapy is necessary with consideration given to withholding or discontinuing diuretic therapy.

Thiazides may decrease serum PBI levels without signs of thyroid disturbance.

ADVERSE REACTIONS

Reserpine

Rauwolfia preparations have caused gastrointestinal reactions including hypersecretion, nausea, vomiting, anorexia, and diarrhea; cardiovascular reactions including angina-like symptoms, arrhythmias (particularly when used concurrently with digitalis or quinidine), and bradycardia; central nervous system reactions including drowsiness, depression, nervousness, paradoxical anxiety, nightmares, rare parkinsonian syndrome and other extrapyramidal tract symptoms, and CNS sensitization manifested by dull sensorium, deafness, glaucoma, uveitis, and optic atrophy. Nasal congestion is a frequent occurrence. Pruritus, rash, dryness of mouth, dizziness, headache, dyspnea, syncope, epistaxis, purpura and other hematologic reactions, impotence or decreased libido, dysuria, muscular aches, conjunctival injection, weight gain, breast engorgement, pseudolactation, and gynecomastia have been reported. These reactions are usually reversible and disappear after the drug is discontinued.

Water retention with edema in patients with hypertensive vascular disease may occur rarely, but the condition generally clears with cessation of therapy or with the administration of a diuretic agent.

Hydralazine

Adverse reactions with hydralazine are usually reversible when dosage is reduced. However, in some cases it may be necessary to discontinue the drug.

Common: Headache, palpitations, anorexia, nausea, vomiting, diarrhea, tachycardia, angina pectoris

Less Frequent: Nasal congestion; flushing; lacrimation; conjunctivitis; peripheral neuritis, evidenced by paresthesias, numbness, and tingling; edema; dizziness, tremors; muscle cramps; psychotic reactions characterized by depression, disorientation, or anxiety; hypersensitivity (including rash, urticaria, pruritus, fever, chills, arthralgia, eosinophilia, and, rarely, hepatitis); constipation; difficulty in micturition; dyspnea; paralytic ileus; lymphadenopathy; splenomegaly; blood dyscrasias, consisting of reduction in hemoglobin and red cell count, leukopenia, agranulocytosis, and purpura; hypotension; paradoxical pressor response.

Hydrochlorothiazide

Gastrointestinal: Anorexia, gastric irritation, nausea, vomiting, cramping, diarrhea, constipation, jaundice (intrahepatic cholestatic), pancreatitis

Central Nervous System: Dizziness, vertigo, paresthesias, headache, xanthopsia

Dermatologic-Hypersensitivity: Purpura, photosensitivity, rash, urticaria, necrotizing angiitis, Stevens-Johnson syndrome, and other hypersensitivity reactions

Hematologic: Leukopenia, thrombocytopenia, agranulocytosis, aplastic anemia

Cardiovascular: Orthostatic hypotension may occur and may be potentiated by alcohol, barbiturates, or narcotics

Other: Hyperglycemia, glycosuria, hyperuricemia, muscle spasm, weakness, restlessness

Whenever adverse reactions are moderate or severe, thiazide dosage should be reduced or therapy withdrawn.

DOSAGE AND ADMINISTRATION

As determined by individual titration (see box warning). Usual dosage is 1 to 2 tablets t.i.d.

Since the antihypertensive effects of reserpine are not immediately apparent, maximal reduction in blood pressure from a given dosage may not occur for 2 weeks. For maintenance, adjust dosage to lowest patient requirement.

When necessary, more potent antihypertensives may be added gradually in dosages reduced by at least 50 percent. Watch effects carefully.

OVERDOSAGE

Reserpine

Signs and Symptoms

Impairment of consciousness may occur and may range from drowsiness to coma, depending upon the severity of overdosage. Flushing of the skin, conjunctival injection, and pupillary constriction are to be expected. Hypotension, hypothermia, central respiratory depression, and bradycardia may develop in cases of severe overdosage. Diarrhea may also occur.

Treatment

Evacuate stomach contents, taking adequate precautions against aspiration and for protection of the airway; instill activated charcoal slurry.

Treat the effects of reserpine overdosage symptomatically. If hypotension is severe enough to require treatment with a vasopressor, use one having a direct action upon vascular smooth muscle (*eg* phenylephrine, levarterenol, metaraminol). Since reserpine is long-acting, observe the patient carefully for at least 72 hours, administering treatment as required.

Hydralazine

Signs and Symptoms

Hypotension, tachycardia, headache and generalized skin flushing are to be expected. Myocardial ischemia and cardiac arrhythmia can develop; profound shock can occur in severe overdosage.

Treatment

Evacuate gastric contents, taking adequate precautions against aspiration and for protection of the airway; instill activated charcoal slurry, if general conditions permit. These manipulations may have to be omitted or carried out after cardiovascular status has been stabilized, since they might precipitate cardiac arrhythmias or increase the depth of shock.

Support of the cardiovascular system is of primary importance. Shock should be treated with volume expanders without resorting to use of vasopressors, if possible. If a vasopressor is required, use one that is least likely to precipitate or aggravate cardiac arrhythmia. Digitalization may be necessary. Renal function must be monitored and supported as required.

No experience has been reported with extracorporeal or peritoneal dialysis.

Hydrochlorothiazide

Signs and Symptoms

Diuresis is to be expected; lethargy of varying degree may appear and may progress to coma within a few hours, with minimal depression of respiration and cardiovascular function and without significant serum electrolyte changes or dehydration. The mechanism of CNS depression with thiazide overdosage is unknown.

GI irritation and hypermotility may occur; temporary elevation of BUN has been reported and serum electrolyte changes could occur, especially in patients with impairment of renal function.

Treatment

Evacuate gastric contents but take care to prevent aspiration, especially in the stuporous or comatose patient. GI effects are usually of short duration, but may require symptomatic treatment.

Monitor serum electrolyte levels and renal function; institute supportive measures as required individually to maintain hydration, electrolyte balance, respiration and cardiovascular-renal function.

HOW SUPPLIED

Tablets (dark salmon pink, dry-coated), each containing 0.1 mg reserpine, 25 mg hydralazine hydrochloride, and 15 mg hydrochlorothiazide; bottles of 30, 60, 100 and 1000.

REV. 5/75

Serpasil®

(reserpine USP)

Tablets Elixir

DESCRIPTION

Reserpine, a pure crystalline alkaloid of rauwolfia, is a white or pale buff to slightly yellowish crystalline powder which darkens slowly on exposure to light and is insoluble in water. Chemically, it is methyl-0-(3,4,5-trimethoxybenzoyl)-reserpate.

ACTIONS

Serpasil probably produces its antihypertensive effects through depletion of tissue stores of catecholamines (epinephrine and norepinephrine) from peripheral sites. This depression of sympathetic nerve function results in a decreased heart rate and a lowering of arterial blood pressure. In contrast, Serpasil's sedative and tranquilizing properties are thought to be related to depletion of 5-hydroxytryptamine from the brain.

Serpasil, like other rauwolfia compounds, is characterized by slow onset of action and sustained effects. Both cardiovascular and central nervous system effects may persist for a period of time following withdrawal of the drug.

INDICATIONS

Mild essential hypertension; also useful as adjunctive therapy with other antihypertensive agents in the more severe forms of hypertension; relief of symptoms in agitated psychotic states (*eg,* schizophrenia), primarily in those individuals unable to tolerate phenothiazine derivatives or those who also require antihypertensive medication.

CONTRAINDICATIONS

Known hypersensitivity, mental depression (especially with suicidal tendencies), active peptic ulcer, ulcerative colitis, and patients receiving electroconvulsive therapy.

WARNINGS

Extreme caution should be exercised in treating patients with a history of mental depression. Discontinue the drug at first sign of despondency, early morning insomnia, loss of appetite, impotence, or self-deprecation. Drug-induced depression may persist for several months after drug withdrawal and may be severe enough to result in suicide.

MAO inhibitors should be avoided or used with extreme caution.

Usage in Pregnancy

The safety of reserpine for use during pregnancy or lactation has not been established; therefore, the drug should be used in pregnant patients or in women of childbearing potential only when, in the judgment of the physician, it is essential to the welfare of the patient. Increased respiratory tract secretions, nasal congestion, cyanosis, and anorexia may occur in neonates and breast-fed infants of reserpine-treated mothers since reserpine crosses the placental barrier and also appears in maternal breast milk.

PRECAUTIONS

Since Serpasil increases gastrointestinal motility and secretion, it should be used cautiously in patients with a history of peptic ulcer, ulcerative colitis, or gallstones (biliary colic may be precipitated).

Caution should be exercised when treating hypertensive patients with renal insufficiency since they adjust poorly to lowered blood pressure levels.

Use Serpasil cautiously with digitalis and quinidine since cardiac arrhythmias have occurred with rauwolfia preparations.

Preoperative withdrawal of reserpine does not assure that circulatory instability will not occur. It is important that the anesthesiologist be aware of the patient's drug intake and consider this in the overall management, since hypotension has occurred in patients receiving rauwolfia preparations. Anticholinergic and/or adrenergic drugs (*eg*, metaraminol, norepinephrine) have been employed to treat adverse vagocirculatory effects.

ADVERSE REACTIONS

Rauwolfia preparations have caused gastrointestinal reactions including hypersecretion, nausea, vomiting, anorexia, and diarrhea; cardiovascular reactions including angina-like symptoms, arrhythmias (particularly when used concurrently with digitalis or quinidine), bradycardia; central nervous system reactions including drowsiness, depression, nervousness, paradoxical anxiety, nightmares, rare parkinsonian syndrome and other extrapyramidal tract symptoms, and CNS sensitization manifested by dull sensorium, deafness, glaucoma, uveitis, and optic atrophy. Nasal congestion is a frequent occurrence. Pruritus, rash, dryness of mouth, dizziness, headache, dyspnea, syncope, epistaxis, purpura and other hematologic reactions, impotence or decreased libido, dysuria, muscular aches, conjunctival injection, weight gain, breast engorgement, pseudolactation, and gynecomastia have been reported. These reactions are usually reversible and usually disappear after the drug is discontinued.

Water retention with edema in patients with hypertensive vascular disease may occur rarely, but the condition generally clears with cessation of therapy or with the administration of a diuretic agent.

DOSAGE AND ADMINISTRATION

For Hypertension: In the average patient not receiving other antihypertensive agents, the usual initial dose is 0.5 mg daily for 1 or 2 weeks. For maintenance, reduce to 0.1 mg to 0.25 mg daily. Higher doses should be used cautiously, because serious mental depression and other side effects may be increased considerably.

For Psychiatric Disorders: The usual initial dose is 0.5 mg, with a range of 0.1 mg to 1.0 mg. Adjust dosage upward or downward according to the patient's response.

Concomitant use of Serpasil with ganglionic blocking agents, guanethidine, veratrum, hydralazine, methyldopa, chlorthalidone, or thiazides necessitates careful titration of dosage with each agent.

OVERDOSAGE

Signs and Symptoms

Impairment of consciousness may occur and may range from drowsiness to coma, depending upon the severity of overdosage. Flushing of the skin, conjunctival injection, and pupillary constriction are to be expected.

Hypotension, hypothermia, central respiratory depression, and bradycardia may develop in cases of severe overdosage. Diarrhea may also occur.

Treatment

Evacuate stomach contents, taking adequate precautions against aspiration and for the protection of the airway; instill activated charcoal slurry.

Treat the effects of reserpine overdosage symptomatically. If hypotension is severe enough to require treatment with a vasopressor, use one having a direct action upon vascular smooth muscle (*eg,* phenylephrine, levarterenol, metaraminol). Since reserpine is long-acting, observe the patient carefully for at least 72 hours, administering treatment as required.

HOW SUPPLIED

Tablets, 1 mg (white, scored); bottles of 100.
Tablets, 0.25 mg (white, scored); bottles of 30, 60, 100, 500, 1000 and 5000.
Tablets, 0.1 mg (white); bottles of 100, 500 and 1000.
Elixir (green, lemon-lime flavored), 0.2 mg per 4-ml teaspoon; bottles of 1 pint.

REV. 5/75

Serpasil®
(reserpine USP)
Parenteral Solution

DESCRIPTION

Reserpine, a pure crystalline alkaloid of rauwolfia, is a white or pale buff to slightly yellowish crystalline powder which darkens slowly on exposure to light and is insoluble in water. Chemically, it is methyl-0-(3,4,5-trimethoxybenzoyl)-reserpate.

ACTIONS

Serpasil probably produces its antihypertensive effects through depletion of tissue stores of catecholamines (epinephrine and norepinephrine) from peripheral sites. This depression of sympathetic nerve function results in a decreased heart rate and a lowering of arterial blood pressure. In contrast, Serpasil's sedative and tranquilizing properties are thought to be related to depletion of 5-hydroxytryptamine from the brain.

Serpasil, like other rauwolfia compounds, is characterized by slow onset of action and sustained effects. Both cardiovascular and central nervous system effects may persist for a period of time following withdrawal of the drug.

INDICATIONS

Hypertensive emergencies, such as acute hypertensive encephalopathy, in which it is desired to reduce blood pressure rapidly; psychiatric conditions only to initiate treatment in those patients unable to accept oral medication or to control symptoms of extreme agitation.

CONTRAINDICATIONS

Known hypersensitivity, mental depression (especially with suicidal tendencies), active peptic ulcer, ulcerative colitis, and patients receiving electroconvulsive therapy.

WARNINGS

Extreme caution should be exercised in treating patients with a history of mental depression. Discontinue the drug at first sign of despondency, early morning insomnia, loss of appetite, impotence, or self-deprecation. Drug-induced depression may persist for several months after drug withdrawal and may be severe enough to result in suicide.

MAO inhibitors should be avoided or used with extreme caution.

Usage in Pregnancy

The safety of reserpine for use during pregnancy or lactation has not been established; therefore, the drug should be used in pregnant patients or in women of child-bearing potential only when, in the judgment of the physician, it is essential to the welfare of the patient. Increased respiratory tract secretions, nasal congestion, cyanosis, and anorexia may occur in neonates and breast-fed infants of reserpine-treated mothers since reserpine crosses the placental barrier and also appears in maternal breast milk.

PRECAUTIONS

Since Serpasil increases gastrointestinal motility and secretion, it should be used cautiously in patients with a history of peptic ulcer, ulcerative colitis, or gallstones (biliary colic may be precipitated).

Caution should be exercised when treating hypertensive patients with renal insufficiency since they adjust poorly to lowered blood pressure levels.

Use Serpasil cautiously with digitalis and quinidine since cardiac arrhythmias have occurred with rauwolfia preparations.

Preoperative withdrawal of reserpine does not assure that circulatory instability will not occur. It is important that the anesthesiologist be aware of the patient's drug intake and consider this in the overall management, since hypotension has occurred in patients receiving rauwolfia preparations. Anti-cholinergic and/or adrenergic drugs (*eg*, metaraminol, norepinephrine) have been employed to treat adverse vagocirculatory effects.

ADVERSE REACTIONS

Rauwolfia preparations have caused gastro-intestinal reactions including hypersecretion, nausea, vomiting, anorexia, and diarrhea; cardiovascular reactions including angina-like symptoms, arrhythmias (particularly when used concurrently with digitalis or quinidine), bradycardia; central nervous system reactions including drowsiness, depression, nervousness, paradoxical anxiety, nightmares, rare parkinsonian syndrome and other extra-pyramidal tract symptoms, and CNS sensitization manifested by dull sensorium, deafness, glaucoma, uveitis, and optic atrophy. Nasal congestion is a frequent occurrence. Pruritus, rash, dryness of mouth, dizziness, headache, dyspnea, syncope, epistaxis, purpura and other hematologic reactions, impotence or decreased libido, dysuria, muscular aches, conjunctival injection, weight gain, breast engorgement, pseudo-lactation, and gynecomastia have been reported. These reactions are usually reversible and usually disappear after the drug is discontinued.

Water retention with edema in patients with hypertensive vascular disease may occur rarely, but the condition generally clears with cessation of therapy or with the administration of a diuretic agent.

DOSAGE AND ADMINISTRATION

Serpasil may be administered intramuscularly in the short-term treatment of hypertensive crises. Because of the varying responsiveness, a titration procedure should be used. An initial dose of 0.5 to 1 mg intramuscularly is followed at intervals of 3 hours, if necessary, by doses of 2 and 4 mg until the blood pressure falls to the desired level. If the 4-mg dose is ineffective, other antihypertensive agents should be used. An initial dose larger than 0.5 mg may induce severe hypotension, particularly in patients with cerebral hemorrhage.

Serpasil may be administered intra-muscularly in psychiatric emergencies to initiate treatment in those patients unable to accept oral medication or to control extreme agitation. The usual dose is from 2.5 mg to 5.0 mg, following a small initial dose to test patient responsiveness.

Concomitant use of Serpasil with ganglionic blocking agents, guanethidine, veratrum, hydralazine, methyldopa, chlorthalidone, or thiazides necessitates careful titration of dosage with each agent.

OVERDOSAGE

Signs and Symptoms

Impairment of consciousness may occur and may range from drowsiness to coma, depending upon the severity of overdosage. Flushing of the skin, conjunctival injection, and pupillary constriction are to be expected. Hypotension, hypothermia, central respiratory depression, and bradycardia may develop in cases of severe overdosage. Diarrhea may also occur.

Treatment

Hypotension is likely to require major therapeutic attention. If a vasopressor is necessary, use one having a direct action upon vascular smooth muscle (*eg*, phenylephrine, levarterenol, metaraminol).

If bradycardia becomes marked, especially with cardiac arrhythmia, consider use of vagal blocking agents along with other appropriate measures.

Treat other effects of reserpine overdosage symptomatically. Since reserpine is long-acting, observe the patient carefully for at least 72 hours, administering treatment as required.

HOW SUPPLIED

Parenteral Solution: Each ml contains 2.5 mg reserpine, 0.1 ml dimethylacetamide, 10 mg adipic acid, 0.1 mg versene, 0.01 ml benzyl alcohol, 0.05 ml polyethylene glycol, 0.5 mg ascorbic acid, and 0.1 mg sodium sulfite in water. *Ampuls,* 2 ml; cartons of 5. *Multiple-dose Vials,* 10 ml; cartons of 1, boxes of 6.

REV. 2/74

Slow-K® (potassium chloride) slow-release tablets

DESCRIPTION

Slow-K is a sugar-coated (not enteric-coated) tablet containing 600 mg potassium chloride (equivalent to 8 mEq) in a wax matrix. This formulation is intended to provide a controlled release of potassium from the matrix to minimize the likelihood of producing high localized concentrations of potassium within the gastrointestinal tract.

ACTIONS

Potassium ion is the principal intracellular cation of most body tissues. Potassium ions participate in a number of essential physiological processes, including the maintenance of intracellular tonicity, the transmission of nerve impulses, the contraction of cardiac, skeletal, and smooth muscle and the maintenance of normal renal function.

Potassium depletion may occur whenever the rate of potassium loss through renal excretion and/or loss from the gastrointestinal tract exceeds the rate of potassium intake. Such depletion usually develops slowly as a consequence of prolonged therapy with oral diuretics, primary or secondary hyperaldosteronism, diabetic ketoacidosis, severe diarrhea, or inadequate replacement of potassium in patients on prolonged parenteral nutrition. Potassium depletion due to these causes is usually accompanied by a concomitant deficiency of chloride and is manifested by hypokalemia and metabolic alkalosis. Potassium depletion may produce weakness, fatigue, disturbances of cardiac rhythm (primarily ectopic beats), prominent U-waves in the electrocardiogram, and in advanced cases flaccid paralysis and/or impaired ability to concentrate urine.

Potassium depletion associated with metabolic alkalosis is managed by correcting the fundamental cause of the deficiency whenever possible and administering supplemental potassium chloride, in the form of high potassium food or potassium chloride solution or tablets.

In rare circumstances (*eg*, patients with renal tubular acidosis) potassium depletion may be associated with metabolic acidosis and hyperchloremia. In such patients potassium replacement should be accomplished with potassium salts other than the chloride, such as potassium bicarbonate, potassium citrate, or potassium acetate.

INDICATIONS

Slow-K is indicated for the treatment of potassium depletion in patients with hypokalemia and metabolic alkalosis, and for the treatment of digitalis intoxication. During therapy serum potassium levels should be monitored and the dosage titrated to achieve the desired clinical and laboratory effects.

Slow-K is also indicated for the prevention of potassium depletion when the dietary intake of potassium is inadequate for this purpose. The prophylactic administration of potassium ion may be indicated in patients receiving digitalis and diuretics for the treatment of congestive heart failure, hepatic cirrhosis with ascites, patients with hypertension on long-term diuretic therapy, hyperaldosteronism states with normal renal function, the nephrotic syndrome, and certain diarrheal states.

CONTRAINDICATIONS

Potassium supplements are contraindicated in patients with hyperkalemia since a further increase in serum potassium concentration in such patients can produce cardiac arrest. Hyperkalemia may complicate any of the following conditions: chronic renal failure, systemic acidosis such as diabetic acidosis, acute dehydration, extensive tissue breakdown as in severe burns, adrenal insufficiency, or the administration of a potassium-sparing diuretic (*eg,* spironolactone, triamterene).

Wax-matrix potassium chloride preparations have produced esophageal ulceration in certain cardiac patients with esophageal compression due to enlarged left atrium.

All solid dosage forms of potassium supplements are contraindicated in any patient in whom there is cause for arrest or delay in tablet passage through the gastrointestinal tract. In these instances, potassium supplementation should be with a liquid preparation.

WARNINGS

In patients with impaired mechanisms for excreting potassium, the administration of potassium salts can produce hyperkalemia and cardiac arrest. This occurs most commonly in patients given potassium by the intravenous route but may also occur in patients given potassium orally. Potentially fatal hyperkalemia can develop rapidly and be asymptomatic. The use of potassium salts in patients with chronic renal disease, or any other condition which impairs potassium excretion, requires particularly careful monitoring of the serum potassium concentration and appropriate dosage adjustment.

Hypokalemia should not be treated by the concomitant administration of potassium salts and a potassium-sparing diuretic (*eg,* spironolactone or triamterene), since the simultaneous administration of these agents can produce severe hyperkalemia.

Potassium chloride tablets have produced stenotic and/or ulcerative lesions of the small bowel and deaths. These lesions are caused by a high localized concentration of potassium ion in the region of a rapidly dissolving tablet, which injures the bowel wall and thereby produces obstruction, hemorrhage, or perforation. Slow-K is a wax-matrix tablet formulated to provide a controlled rate of release of potassium chloride and thus to minimize the possibility of a high local concentration of potassium ion near the bowel wall. While the reported frequency of small bowel lesions is much less with wax-matrix tablets (less than one per 100,000 patient-years) than with enteric-coated potassium chloride tablets (40-50 per 100,000 patient-years), a few cases associated with wax-matrix tablets have been reported. These data are from foreign marketing experience. Slow-K should be discontinued immediately and the possibility of bowel obstruction or perforation considered if severe vomiting, abdominal pain, distention, or gastrointestinal bleeding occurs.

Hypokalemia in patients with metabolic *acidosis* should be treated with an alkalinizing potassium salt such as potassium bicarbonate, potassium citrate, or potassium acetate.

PRECAUTIONS

The diagnosis of potassium depletion is ordinarily made by demonstrating hypokalemia in a patient with a clinical history suggesting some cause for potassium depletion. In interpreting the serum potassium level, the physician should bear in mind that acute alkalosis *per se* can produce hypokalemia in the absence of a deficit in total body potassium, while acute acidosis *per se* can increase the serum potassium concentration into the normal range even in the presence of a reduced total body potassium. The treatment of potassium depletion, particularly in the presence of cardiac disease, renal disease, or acidosis, requires careful attention to acid-base balance and appropriate monitoring of serum electrolytes, the electrocardiogram, and the clinical status of the patient.

ADVERSE REACTIONS

The most common adverse reactions to oral potassium salts are nausea, vomiting, abdominal discomfort, and diarrhea. These symptoms are due to irritation of the gastrointestinal tract and are best managed by diluting the preparation further, taking the dose with meals, or reducing the dose.

The most severe adverse effects are hyperkalemia (see Contraindications, Warnings and Overdosage) and gastrointestinal obstruction, bleeding, or perforation (see Warnings).

OVERDOSAGE

The administration of oral potassium salts to persons with normal excretory mechanisms for potassium rarely causes serious hyperkalemia. However, if excretory mechanisms are impaired or if potassium is administered too rapidly intravenously, potentially fatal hyperkalemia can result (see Contraindications and Warnings). It is important to recognize that hyperkalemia is usually asymptomatic and may be manifested only by an increased serum potassium concentration and characteristic electrocardiographic changes (peaking of T-waves, loss of P-wave depression of S-T segment, and prolongation of the QT interval). Late manifestations include muscle paralysis and cardiovascular collapse from cardiac arrest.

Treatment measures for hyperkalemia include the following: (1) elimination of foods and medications containing potassium and of potassium-sparing diuretics; (2) intravenous administration of 300 to 500 ml/hr of 10% dextrose solution containing 10-20 units of insulin per 1,000 ml; (3) correction of acidosis, if present, with intravenous sodium bicarbonate; (4) use of exchange resins, hemodialysis, or peritoneal dialysis.

In treating hyperkalemia, it should be recalled that in patients who have been stabilized on digitalis, too rapid a lowering of the serum potassium concentration can produce digitalis toxicity.

DOSAGE AND ADMINISTRATION

The usual dietary intake of potassium by the average adult is 40 to 80 mEq per day. Potassium depletion sufficient to cause hypokalemia usually requires the loss of 200 or more mEq of potassium from the total body store.

Dosage must be adjusted to the individual needs of each patient but is typically in the range of 20 mEq per day for the prevention of hypokalemia to 40-100 mEq per day or more for the treatment of potassium depletion.

HOW SUPPLIED

Tablets (pale orange, sugar-coated), each containing 600 mg potassium chloride (equivalent to 8 mEq); bottles of 100 and 1000.

REV. 7/75

CIBA Pharmaceutical Company
Division of CIBA-GEIGY Corporation
Summit, New Jersey 07901

PRINTED IN U.S.A. SEPTEMBER 1975 D/00/5529A 15